Beating My Breast

Kate Cramond grew up on an orchard in South Australia, and fondly remembers climbing trees and pelting her brothers and sisters with apples. At university she studied biological sciences, in between bushwalking, climbing mountains and driving all over the place. After that, she settled into an assortment of environmental jobs, in between writing stories, marrying and raising two awesome daughters. Getting breast cancer wasn't exactly on her to do list, but it did give her plenty to write about. She hopes her words will help others (and make her many confessions worthwhile ☺).

Kate Cramond

Beating My Breast

A diary of life and connection

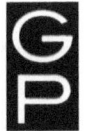

Beating My Breast: A diary of life and connection
ISBN 978 1 76041 769 7
Copyright © Kate Cramond 2019
Cover artwork: Tabitha Stowe

First published 2019 by
GINNINDERRA PRESS
PO Box 3461 Port Adelaide 5015
www.ginninderrapress.com.au

Preface

How wonderful it is, being able to write again. These last few weeks I've felt it trickling back to me: my mental zing.

I lost it after the first round of chemo. For months I was dull like tarnished silver, unable to read newspapers or follow documentaries – let alone remember a sentence I'd just read or heard. It was bad.

But not as bad as having cancer huh?

I like to think of this diary as the final round of my treatment. A purging of the whole process: both awful and amazing – all of it. Whatever springs to mind on the day is what you'll get.

So come along for the ride and see where this takes me.

1 September 2014

I've been sliding for a while. Bits of me scraping off, rocks bouncing around me, panic in my head. The scree slope got me nearly a year ago. One in eight Australian women get breast cancer in their lifetime. An ordinary statistic: that's me.

Since going through my treatment, I've felt a weight on my shoulders like an invisible hump. It nudges at me when I sit in the car, irritates me as I sleep. I need to offload. Or reload. I need *something* because at the moment there's a greyness in my soul. Why can't I shake myself off and get on with things? After all, the sun's shining, it's the first day of spring. But I was diagnosed in the last month of spring, so the sunshine, buzzy bees and blooming flowers didn't protect me.

Ah, you see where I'm at, don't you?

I'm better now. Or at least I should be, statistically. But I've never felt worse. I'd like to say I'm at rock bottom but the scree is still rumbling beneath me.

When I think of rocks and screes, I think of bushwalking. That was me, once. Tanned, fit, capable – striding along with my backpack rubbing welts into my shoulders. I can see why older people return to their youth in their memories. The luxury of being unencumbered, oh yes that's appealing.

Ha, don't kid yourself, oldies. In youth, the rocks are already piling up in metaphorical backpacks.

*

I spent nearly every holiday during my university years going on long bushwalks with friends. We left our books behind, squashed ourselves and our heavy packs into cars and headed for the great outdoors. I loved it.

In my third year of university, I started asking my younger brother to come along too. I'm not sure why he wanted to hang out with a ragtag bunch of students all intent on showing off their knowledge but I guess he was like me – he loved being out bush, away from the confines of ordinary life.

So he came with us on a walk to a place called Edeowie Gorge. The hike started with a bit of a huff and puff over a low pass to the pound, an elevated plain ringed by mountains. Then it was an easy walk through open woodlands to the opposite end of the pound, where a creek cut down through a spectacular gorge. I can't remember the details, but at some point along the gorge we came to the top of a waterfall. At that time of year, the creek was just a trickle, but when the water dribbled over the edge and sprayed into infinity…oh my.

We stood near the edge, staring at sheer cliffs coloured ochre by the late afternoon sun and the shadowy creek bed lined with trees far below. One of the guys picked up a pebble and tossed it over. The sharp crack as it hit rock startled a pair of cockatoos, who took to the air with raucous shrieks. I've always loved that sound. Although it makes me sad too, just a little.

The next morning, we found the descent route, a traverse off to the left of the waterfall. The hardest bit was protected by a rope bolted to the rock, and we clung to this and sidled along with our backpacks tugging us towards the abyss. I wasn't scared, back then.

Once off the narrow ledge, it got easier, but now there was no rope. It was steep going, with nothing but scrappy bushes to hold onto. My brother Michael and a couple of other guys were below, out of sight, but I could still hear them.

'Be careful,' shouted Ben. 'There's a bit of drop here. Why don't you hand me your pack?'

'Okay,' shouted Michael, then silence.

Then a cry of surprise, a crashing, bouncing noise, a pause – then a loud thud. At the bottom of the waterfall.

I screamed.

My legs were scratched and bleeding by the time I reached them.

But Mike was there beside Ben, he was safe! His pack lay far below. Dismayed by the madwoman who was his sister, he tried to disappear into the hillside. I think I might have hugged him, poor guy.

At the bottom, we surveyed the mess. The pack's external frame was bent and the contents splayed across the creek bed. Deep red port was seeping through the canvas fabric like blood. It gave me chills.

Mike pulled out the dripping port bladder with a grin and Ben laughed. 'Oh well, we'd better drink it now.'

As the others settled down on various creek boulders, I got to work on the pack. Mike pretended not to notice as I tipped everything out and spread his underwear and toiletries out for the world to see. I cleaned the port off everything as best I could with manky water from the pool below the waterfall. As I finished straightening the pack frame, I realised I had an audience – everyone was laughing at me. I didn't care.

When finally I'd finished fussing, I sat beside Michael, and it's possible, even likely, that I gave him another hug. He stood abruptly and walked off to have a cigarette.

That's one of the rocks in my backpack.

2 September

It's another glorious spring day. My dog has found a patch of sunshine at my feet and there's a currawong calling from a gumtree across the road. But this morning, like most mornings of late, I woke feeling sad. My hand went to my right breast, the one that had the lump. The lump that is now gone, along with a chunk of my breast. A physical reminder that there's no going back.

Nonetheless, my body is rejuvenating. The strange stiffness in my muscles from radiotherapy is fading, I've put on weight and have a funky hairdo. Somebody I work with said I look like Annie Lennox, woo hoo!

Yes, I'm going back to work. *Going back*…those words make me anxious. If there are any perks from having cancer, Changing Your Life should be one of them. Time to shake off the badness and move with the gladness. Or something like that.

My life changed immediately, sure. I sat around at home for months feeling like crap. My thoughts were muddled, my emotions down the toilet. I became needy, not something that sits well with someone like me.

I'm still needy.

Nature has given us this incredible ability to think and feel and want, but despite our best efforts we're confined by the demands of our bodies. It's just a quirk of physiology that lets us believe that our minds are somehow separate, that we can rise above our chemistry.

Let me tell you about chemotherapy, just to prove my point.

*

Three weeks after my breast surgery, I went to see my oncologist (cancer doctor) to find out what treatment I needed next. He was friendly and reassuring, and my hopes rose. He began by typing my statistics into the program used to determine my treatment. Age, family history, medical history, type of cancer, stage of cancer (aggressiveness) and grade of cancer (spread). My cancer was moderately aggressive, and had spread from my breast to two lymph nodes under my arm. Stage 2, grade 2.

He said that at forty-seven I was considered 'young' for a breast cancer person. Tell a middle-aged woman she's young, even when she's got cancer, and what do you get? I smiled.

As the computer did its computing, he explained that treatment options were too complex these days for an individual to make an assessment. His gaze returned to his computer screen and he paused, tapping his pen.

My heart began to pound.

When he looked up with his expression ready, I knew the outcome. Chemotherapy. The one thing I wanted to avoid at all costs. Of course, I didn't *have* to have it. Nobody could force me.

Enter the statistics. My doctor explained that according to his program my ten-year survival rate would improve with each treatment as follows:

- surgery plus radiation therapy to the right breast = 67%
- chemotherapy = +9%
- hormonal therapy (after active treatment was finished) = +13%.

Bringing me to a grand total of 89%. Nearly 90%, wow – a winning equation! A great result!

He explained that if the benefits of chemo had been less than 5%, it might not have been worth the side effects (because we all know chemo is devastating). But for me, at my age, a 9% improvement was worth fighting for. Go for gold!

After chemo, I'd move on to six weeks of radiation therapy, but that was a given – it was standard treatment for women who had lumpectomies (where the tumour and surrounding tissue is removed, rather than the whole breast). Radiation would blitz any lingering cancer cells in my breast.

But chemo was a priority, to make sure any rogue cells invading my body were nuked (my words, not his). He recommended six 'rounds' of a regime called FEC, three weeks apart. I'd heard that some people only had four rounds, so asked why I needed six. The answer? Because I was young to be getting breast cancer (not good), but because of that I had many, many years to live (better). Go for gold, girl.

He said I should start ASAP. It was a shame Christmas was coming but hey – what was more important?

Soon I was staggering out the door clutching a script for antibiotics (because I had a lingering infection under my arm from surgery), with my chemo commencement date ringing in my ears. The eighteenth of December. Only a week away. Exactly one week before Christmas.

The next day, the phone rang. Could I attend a chemotherapy education session at the hospital that afternoon?

There was no hopping off this conveyor belt.

*

At the hospital, a friendly nurse sat me down in a little room away from the wards (where subdued people sat in large chairs with various bits of medical equipment around them). She told me everything I needed to know about FEC. It's a combination of three chemicals: fluorouracil, epirubicin and cyclophosphamide. At the time, this meant nothing to me. Now I feel queasy just typing the names.

These drugs are designed to damage or kill cells in the body while they're dividing. The most active ones that replace themselves frequently are hit hardest: cells in the skin, hair, nails, mucous membranes (digestive tract) and immune system – just for starters. But it's all for a good reason because which cells are the most active of all? Cancer cells, duh! That's all they do – divide, divide, divide. Because of that, not only are they more likely to be damaged by chemo, but they take longer to heal afterwards because most of their energy is invested in reproducing themselves.

With each successive round of chemo, any cancer cells in my body would be progressively damaged and eliminated, while my normal cells would take a hit but recover more quickly. At the end of it all, I would be okay but the cancer wouldn't.

There's one problem here. Nobody could tell me if I had any cancer cells left in my body. My tumour was gone, along with the adjoining lymph nodes – so there was a fair chance I was already clear of cancer. I could be flooding my body with toxic chemicals needlessly.

Without an answer to that problem, the only thing left to do was fall back on those statistics: that chemo would reduce the chances of a person like me dying within ten years by 9%. I couldn't argue with that.

But here's where wishful thinking comes in. I liked to imagine that a fit and generally healthy person like myself would be less likely to be brought down by the drugs. I'd be the good news story. And I believed the chemical effects of my chemo would be short term. In no time, I'd be back to my usual self. Hmm.

So I sat there in my education session as the nurse calmly explained the side effects I could expect. The most immediate one would be nausea, which these days is controllable with drugs. 'Many people feel nothing.' Yay.

I'd also suffer weakened immunity, fatigue and hair loss, and a range of other likely symptoms including digestive problems, damaged skin and nails, skin photo-sensitivity, weight loss/gain, forgetfulness, depression…

There was a cycle of symptoms too. After each dose, I'd feel nauseous and tired for a few days, then after a week my white blood cell count would plummet and I'd be at risk of getting sick (and ending up in Emergency). I'd probably get mouth sores. After two weeks, my head hair would fall out, and in the third week I'd start feeling better and could do some nice things. 'Time to treat yourself!'

Then before I got too healthy, it'd be time to bomb my cells with chemo again. The nurse advised me that timing was critical. I should do everything possible to stay well and avoid delaying any chemo doses.

So I trotted off home with my booklets, my naïve optimism and a little card to present at Emergency if I needed to be admitted.

3 September

It's the third day of spring now. Tick tock, time is passing. I've been drifting, not just for the ten months since my diagnosis, but for years. I blinked – forgive the cliché – and twenty years passed. Why have I let this happen?

I'm sure for me the answer lies partly in that load of rocks, slowing my tread, dulling my passion.

The other night, I watched a BBC documentary called *The Power of the Placebo*. In one experiment, a young guy was taken to the top of the Italian Alps and asked to walk thirty minutes with an oxygen tank. He wasn't told the tank didn't actually contain oxygen. Nonetheless, his performance improved markedly. His body responded to the placebo oxygen as if it were actual oxygen: the same chemical pathways were stimulated. He believed the 'oxygen' would help him, so it did.

If I'd really believed I could heal my own cancer, is it possible I could have? That way of thinking isn't new to me, but when faced with my own mortality and the promises of modern medicine, it was a no-brainer. I jumped on the medical treatment train. No, what concerns me more is the reverse scenario: did the power of my thinking, the quality of my thinking, make me a more likely cancer candidate? Or is that just hippy gaga stuff designed to make me feel guilty?

There's no doubt that thoughts and body are not separate. My thinking produces physiological responses, whether I'm aware of them or not. I'm reminded of this every day. My treatment has pushed me into menopause, and everyone knows what that means…hot flushes. Joy of joys. They come erratically and without warning, except in one situation. All I have to do is think of something that upsets me and the heat floods through me. My emotions, so closely linked to thoughts, are a trigger.

This leads me to one of my pet topics. In the same way that emotions trigger a physiological response, memories can do the same. Think back to a traumatic time in your life and feel the quickening in your body as it replays the stress. Some people argue that we squirrel away emotions with our memories, and these emotions can weigh us down (the negative ones anyway – surely a memory-load of happiness and laughter can't be a problem?). So, by letting ourselves relive these negative memories, we can let the emotions rush out. Go free! Fly away, sadness, badness and shame.

It does work, on some levels. I've tried a few techniques over the years and felt the tingling flow of energy out of me. It feels like a release.

Try this exercise, which comes from my reading about mindfulness. Lie down, get comfy and breathe slowly and deeply. Now run your awareness over your body and scan for tense or painful spots. Focus your attention on one of these areas and breathe into it. Keep breathing and notice what you feel or think.

Often when I do this, I feel a rising tension in my body, a tightness in my chest. Odd feelings or memories can pop up and surprise me. As

I continue breathing, this emotional intensity peaks and then subsides to nothing. Whoosh! Gone. Then I move onto the next spot.

It's a lovely exercise. Afterwards I feel lighter, calmer. Does that mean the tense areas have been holding onto those feelings or memories all that time? I can't say, but it's fascinating.

But does it help me when I come back to the present? Am I better able to face the world? The evidence isn't convincing so far.

One thing I'm sure of. The body stores memories as much as the mind, and with a tighter grip. Think of it this way. If an experience causes physical stress or trauma, surely it's plausible that a residue of this stress remains in the affected parts of the body? A kind of physical memory.

I reckon my body is a treasure trove.

I'm a jaw clencher. A teeth gritter. And I'm thinking there's a story in every ridge and fracture in my teeth. So here goes…close my eyes, focus on my jaw – breathe, breathe.

Aha! I'm trapped in a sleeping bag with two of my older brothers sitting on the opening. It's hot and I can't breathe properly, I'm shouting and crying. I'm really upset, dammit! But they don't listen, they don't care.

This memory isn't new to me, but the intensity of the experience is. If I'd told someone about it yesterday, I'd have laughed and felt nothing. But today, when I let my jaw do the talking, the result is quite different.

It's just a small example. I'm not blaming those brothers who did that to me (yeah, right!), but it seems that my jaw hasn't forgotten. And who can say if my mild claustrophobia came before the sleeping bag incidents or after…

Let's try my teeth. Hmm, easy.

'Bucky, bucky beaver!' chanted the boys as we mucked around on the lawn after school (no need to name the culprits). I walked away, pretending not to care, but the sourness was in my belly, the frustration in my fists.

It was true. I had buck teeth – big lovely white front teeth that stuck out, just a bit. All straightened now, at my parents' expense, but for a while I was terribly self-conscious. I've a photo of me in my early teens, standing on the back lawn in the sunshine. Blue eyes, cute smile, long hair streaked with sun…but what catches my eyes when I look at the photo? Those teeth.

4 September

Surely there are some good memories buried in my physical past?

Hmm, I'm focusing on my right little toe.

High school. My Year 12 end of year dance. We didn't do formals at my school, or in most schools as far as I can remember. This was, after all, back in the olden days – as my kids so charmingly call them.

My school had ballroom dances to celebrate stuff, which was a bit old-fashioned even for back then. The Catholic boys college down the road provided us with partners to dance with. ('Tis true, I went to an all-girls school. But sadly I wasn't one of those wild Catholic girls. Nope. I liked horses and climbing trees.)

Because of my love of roaming around barefoot in summer, I had wide feet. Sturdy feet, but not pretty. So, on this long-awaited night, I squeezed them into pointy-toed high heels. Blue shoes to match my new blue dress.

Like most girls my age, I thought I was ugly. Pimples, braces, fat bum – that was me. But on this night something was different. I'd finished my exams and knew I'd done well. One of my older brothers (who all my friends thought was a hunk) had dropped me off in his hotted up Datsun SSS, and I'd already started learning to drive. The night was warm, and I felt something thawing in me.

I'd had my eyes on a guy who was often at my bus stop after school. We never talked, of course. I was shy. But as soon as I walked into the hall, there he was, asking me to dance. Mary Cousins was right beside me in a gorgeous lacy dress, smelling of expensive perfume, and yet he picked me.

After a few sentences, we ran out of things to say. We stumbled through the foxtrot and moved on to an awkward waltz. His hands were sweaty and his breath sour with nerves. Up close, his acne was even worse than mine. I felt mean, but I couldn't wait to get away.

On my way back from the ladies' room, my friend Anne grabbed my arm. 'Come outside,' she said, pulling me through the side doors.

A guy met my eyes as soon as walked outside. He was tall, olive-skinned. I didn't talk to him, but when I went back inside he followed me. And he asked me to dance.

The frumpy ballroom dancing phase of the evening was finished, and Kim Wilde's 'Kids in America' blasted through the speakers. Everyone poured onto the dance floor, cheering. Five or six songs later, the lights dimmed further and Spandau Ballet's 'True' came on. My guy took me in his arms and we swayed together, our hearts beating fast. As the music faded, he lifted my chin and we kissed. Back then, I'm sad to say, I read lots of romance novels, and this was definitely a Mills & Boons moment.

Funny thing is, I can't remember what happened after that. All I can say is I didn't see him again, and it didn't matter. A gorgeous guy had kissed me. Me! Braces, pimples and all. I was in heaven.

But the next day I could barely walk. My right little toe had an enormous blister and my feet felt like they'd been mangled.

Those damned blue shoes.

5 September

All this dredging up of my youth has stirred my subconscious. I keep getting flashes of feeling that connect me to myself. Old me, young me. Is the young me still living on, rarely recognised but still having her say? That outdoorsy girl who dreamed of adventure – oh, where is she?

Perhaps she really was just a figment of youth, caught up in the promise of a life not yet lived. A stage in my evolution on the way to adulthood, swept up in teenage hormones and way too many fantasy and romance novels.

But there's something wonderful in that process when your mind starts stretching at its leash. When you're still a kid but feeling the tendrils of possibility. Is this me? Can my life be like this?

I felt that stretching in Year 11. Before then I was caught in my tight world of school, year after year, and the difficulties of teenage social life. Or in my case, lack of social life. I was stranded on a farm in the hills on weekends and, although I liked my horsey friends, they weren't where the action was happening. School was the place where I needed to fit in.

But sometime in Year 11, when I was fourteen going on fifteen, these concerns started to drop away. I still hated my body and obsessed about food and dieting. My eyes still followed the popular girls around, coveting their charmed lives. But nonetheless, I found myself inexplicably happier.

Until in early Year 12 something happened that made my world close in on me. There's a song from that time that brings it all back: 'Harden My Heart' by Quarterflash. It's not the words that stick with me, it's the saxophone and relentless drums pulling me out of childhood into a world that would never be the same again.

My nephew died. I mention this not because I want sympathy, but because he deserves to be remembered doesn't he? There's nothing sadder than a bright life, snuffed early and then slowly forgotten. He's in my photo album too. Near my bucky beaver photo is one of him astride my dad's vintage motorbike. Even though his feet barely touch the foot pegs, he looks proud of himself. He didn't get to live long enough to worry about stuff like cancer.

I remember my first day back at school after he died. Everything was the same, but changed forever. My classmates' prattle seemed pointless and their sympathy just politeness. How could they understand? But I couldn't understand either. It made no sense, this being alive when others were no longer. Where was Simeon? How could he just be gone?

Gone. The loneliness of that word.

Who am I to worry when at least I'm still alive?

8 September

I forgot to finish writing about my chemo experience, which is ironic since it's chemo that has made me so forgetful. Ah, the joys.

On 18 December, I stood at the hospital admission desk as they clipped on my wrist tag. Already I was numb.

The actual process of administering my chemotherapy was fairly mundane. But horrific. Already I feel the sickness in my gut, reliving it.

I was seated in a large, reclining chair with a pillow behind my back and another on my lap. A smiling nurse came over and introduced herself. She placed a bowl of warm water in my lap and put my left hand in it, explaining this was to 'prepare' my veins. (I didn't think about it at the time, but they had to administer chemo through veins in my left arm because my right arm was damaged from the surgery: the removal of lymph nodes in my armpit had weakened my lymphatic system. But more on that later.) Then she offered me a glass of water and a large pill – the first of three anti-nausea drugs. As I swallowed my pill, she explained I'd be given the other two in my intravenous line before starting the chemo.

'Why do I need three?' I asked.

'Oh,' she said blithely, 'these chemo drugs are powerful. Before anti-nausea drugs were available, chemo patients would start vomiting violently as soon as the drugs hit their bloodstream – and it would continue for days. They couldn't leave hospital.' She reached behind a curtain and pulled out a wobbly IV stand. 'Ready?'

No way. I nodded.

She lifted my hand from the bowl, patted it dry and fitted a tourniquet cuff on my forearm. As the veins began to pop out, she stroked one on the back of my hand. 'Ah, this is a good one!' She released the tourniquet then ripped the packaging from a shiny needle.

I looked away. A nurse across the room rewarded me with a big smile as she peeled off her purple gloves.

Once the cannula was in and safely taped to my skin, my nurse connected up the IV line then injected the second anti-nausea drug into a port in the line. She gestured to two bags swinging from the IV stand, their cold contents already trickling into my bloodstream. 'The small one's dexamethasone, a steroid which helps with the nausea, and the other is saline, to keep you hydrated. We don't want the chemicals to get too concentrated do we? Once they're empty, we'll start on the epirubicin.'

Now I got to sit and look around. Another nurse brought me sandwiches and fruit, and I devoured them with sudden hunger. Steroids do that, I've been told. The ward was full, but quiet. Some people had relatives or friends beside them, most didn't. Not everyone had IV lines: some came and went for a brief injection or tablet, others sat patiently as a nurse struggled to find a vein, or cleaned the surgically implanted ports in their neck or upper arm. Most people were older than me, and surprisingly, most had hair. A couple of women appeared to have wigs, and one younger woman breezed through the room with an exuberant arrangement of scarves on her head. It didn't seem possible that in two weeks that could be me.

Interestingly, not many people fitted my stereotype of enfeebled, sickly cancer person. Maybe there was hope for me?

But now my nurse was back with a loaded trolley. She hung a new bag of saline on my IV stand and then perched on a stool with her knees touching mine. 'Are you ready for the red push?' she said brightly.

This was epirubicin, the drug that would make me bald. It came in two oversize syringes and was the colour of red cordial.

'You'll see this in your pee afterwards,' she said, smiling, then moved onto the serious stuff. 'This drug must be syringed slowly into your IV line while being diluted with saline, otherwise it will burn your veins. It will feel uncomfortable but this should help.' She placed a hot pack on my wrist and squeezed my fingers encouragingly. 'If you need another one, let me know.'

Then she commenced Operation Red Push. The red liquid mingled slowly with the saline in the tube, then disappeared into my hand. I felt it going up my arm: cold, damaging, hostile. Now it would be in my heart, spreading through my system in toxic pulses. At war. My head began to feel strange, and my nostrils filled with a fizzing, chemical tang. My forearm began to ache and the nurse popped another hot pack there too.

From then on, things blurred. Another syringe of epi followed by a smaller one of fluorouracil. Finally an IV bag of cyclophosphamine, and one more bag of saline. Done.

A flurry of nurses checked I felt okay, removed my cannula, reminded me to book my next appointment and pointed me towards the toilet. I filled the bowl with brilliant orangey pink urine, then as instructed flushed twice and washed my hands thoroughly. (I needed to flush twice after peeing for a few days after each treatment. This was to protect other people from the chemicals in my urine. Nice, huh?)

My face in the mirror was sallow. I studied my frightened eyes and doomed hair. There was no going back now.

9 September

It was almost interesting, ticking off the side effects that followed.

I went home, had a cool shower (it was 37°C outside) and jumped in bed. It was too hot to snuggle in, but I pulled my sheet over me and accepted tea and cake from my daughter with a smile. This wasn't too bad.

An hour later, I felt a twinge of nausea. I downed a Maxolon pill as instructed and picked up my book again. All good. Within thirty minutes, I was flat on my back on the bare sheet with a wet flannel over my face. The nausea was so bad I could barely speak or move in case I threw up toxic chemo-vomit all over my beautiful bedroom. I stayed like that for hours until a nurse came and gave me a turbocharged injection of Maxolon. As I waited for the nausea to subside, I listened to the nurse talking to my family in hushed tones. I was their patient now; they needed to take their new role seriously.

At last, I felt a bit better and managed to crawl to the toilet for another pink pee, then slither back to bed.

The nausea lingered for days, and the drugs I took for it made me jittery. I was tired but couldn't sleep well, and so vague I lost whole junks of time. My head felt like you could fry eggs on it. My body oscillated between hot and 'boiling over, stop the car!' My limbs were puffy, my digestive system was on strike, my surgery scars ached, my food tasted wrong.

Just as I was beginning to feel more normal, my mouth developed sores which would soon reduce me to eating mush. And on Day 14, bang on target, I pulled out my first clump of head hair. New Year's Eve.

The next day, a friend and my daughter shaved off my hair, and the transformation was complete.

*

That, by the way, was just a taste of the side effects. Which brings me back to why I began describing my chemotherapy in the first place.

We're fooling ourselves thinking we're somehow separate from the chemical processes of our bodies. I was told what would happen during chemo. Then I got the stuff and things happened just as they said it would. My bodily processes were known, definable and generally predictable. In this situation, Kate the Person was much less important than Kate the Conglomeration of Chemical Interactions.

My chemicals did as they were told: my body was meant to be thrashed by the chemo and it was. My healthy cells were collateral damage in a war.

The result? Healthy cells, 1 (millions dead or damaged, but recovering); cancer cells, 0 (all dead and gone). That's the theory. But there are no guarantees. No knowing if I had any cancer cells left in me before treatment. And if I did, there's no knowing if the chemo killed them all. And whatever the outcome, there's no knowing if the cancer will come back.

All I'm left with is hope. The ridiculous belief that I'll be okay. Fat lot of use that's been until now, eh?

Five months after finishing chemo, the effects of those chemicals are still with me. My nails, like rings on a tree trunk, show the damage. Ridges and dips, nearly grown out, make my nails weak and misshapen. My regrowing head hair is no longer a definitive sign, more a suggestion, a maybe. And my body hair, oddly, has grown back longer. It's a temporary stress response, apparently. Anorexics have the same problem.

My white blood cell count is still lower than normal, so my immune system hasn't quite recovered. And my brain? Oh no, let's not go there. If I'm damaged for life, I don't want to know about it.

All of this makes me wonder, more than I ever have, about who I am. The person I've relied on for forty-seven years – is she merely a construct, a chemical concoction? And the sadness I've been feeling, is that just chemicals too? My hormonal therapy drug (the final phase of treatment) pulsing through my system, playing havoc with oestrogen levels wherever it goes?

One day they'll produce chemical formulas that define us as individuals. Oh right, I guess that's DNA, isn't it? Delve back into my biological training and I get AGCT, the four nucleic acids that make up DNA. Adenine, guanine, cytosine, thymine – all arranged in specific sequences. If you map my DNA (gene) sequence, it's unique. Absolutely unique to me. But not unique enough to make me any different to the one in eight women who get breast cancer. Stop pretending you're different, that you're above it all. Jump in and relish the mess. Really?

I'm still waiting for the clean-up.

10 September

On TV last night, after the business news and before the weather, was a segment on a photographic exhibition called *The Scar Project*. It's a kind of breast cancer reality check. I watched the images of women with half breasts, no breasts, one breast, no nipples – their skin cleaved by long scars, many of them puckered and disfiguring. Mostly young women, some sad, some not – a progression of faces, women who didn't see it coming.

But in a funny way it was comforting. All those women, ordinary people, they didn't look like they deserved such a fate. I bet they, too, keep wondering what they did wrong.

*

I catch myself all the time. Stray thoughts sneaking around in the shadows. Why didn't I? Should I have? Was it that?

It's crazy how we punish ourselves in our youth. I didn't like much about myself for a very long time. Those breasts (that I'd do anything to get back now) were high on my list of Not Good Enough features. They were marred by fine stretch marks from all the yo-yo dieting of my teens, and not as shapely as I imagined everyone else's were.

When I had surgery, my breasts were already scarred by life. They'd never recovered their former size after two rounds of pregnancy and breastfeeding, and were way down on the perkiness scale compared to my youth.

But in breast cancer terms I'd mostly done the right things. I had kids. Tick. I breastfed them (for around a year each). Tick, tick. I got pregnant before I turned thirty – but only just. Not really a tick. Although I tried the contraceptive pill, it was only for brief periods when younger. Half a tick.

Perhaps I need to delve deeper. What does a breast symbolise? Nurturing, mothering, loving. When I cry, I feel the pain radiating from my heart, my solar plexus – and my breasts.

Didn't I love myself enough? Was I hurting too much? Did I let others hurt me?

If you map my life as a series of footsteps, are there points where the steps keep returning, stamping out a glowing pathway that screams, 'Here! And here!'? Convergence points where the damage was done. I can't erase those points, if they exist, but I want to recognise them. I can't help it.

*

I don't know why but my thoughts keep going back to rocks. They've featured big time in my life, or at least in my young adult life.

Once, I fancied myself as brave. Tough, even. No doubt this was my way of coping in a large family, or maybe I was just destined to be a bit of a tomboy. Whatever the story, it started coming unstuck when I was in Central Australia after finishing uni. I was doing the Around Australia trip with my friend Tara and it had taken us over a month to get to Alice Springs from Adelaide. We were camping out, taking each day as it comes, living by our instincts and our hearts.

While in Alice, we met up with my old boyfriend Rudy, who was also travelling the inland. He came with us to check out a place called Ndala Gorge. After we set up camp, he came with me on a walk through the gorge, and not far along we decided to climb up the side of the gorge and see what was beyond. As we climbed, it got steeper and rockier, and he veered left looking for an easier ascent.

'Come this way,' he called, but I ignored him.

The cliffy section above me looked scalable, and back then I always had something to prove. Up I went, confident my agility and strength would get me to the top. And it would have too, except a rock came away in my hand and I slipped. I'm not sure how far I fell, at most a couple of metres, but I landed on a rock and my ankle collapsed beneath me. The pain, oh crap.

Rudy heard me fall; he was calling but I couldn't answer. I sat there, crumpled, not moving in case the pain got worse.

'Are you okay?' he yelled, climbing down to me.

I managed to point to my ankle.

'Can you move?'

I shook my head, gasping as a wave of nausea hit me.

He stayed with me for a while, trying to get me to move but I wouldn't. Couldn't.

'I'll go get Tara, she can help get you down.' And he was gone, bounding down the steep slope like a mountain goat.

I must have waited for an hour at least, but I don't remember it. By the time Rudy and Tara appeared, my ankle was swollen and throbbing. They helped me up, and waited as I sucked in air, trying not to vomit. Then slowly, slowly, we made our way down. It was too steep for them to help me much so I had to slither down with my foot held up in front of me, using my arms and bum for support. Near the bottom it got so steep they lowered me down with a rope as I sobbed with pain and fear. Not a glorious moment for me.

The final stretch was fairly easy, so I put my arms around their shoulders and hopped.

An older couple stood watching us, shaking their heads.

'You young people will do stupid things,' the woman said. Like I deserved it.

And wouldn't you know it, I saw that woman again a week or so later in a different camping ground. I hopped into public toilets on my crutches and was surrounded by tut-tutting women. When I told them what had happened, they nodded sympathetically, and the woman in question exclaimed, 'Oh, you poor dear, that must have been awful.' Really. A nice study in human nature, don't you think? (Just an aside.)

Cut to a year or so later, when I was on a five-day bushwalking trip in the Grampians. If you've been there, you'll know how incredible the rocks are. Lots of sandstone shaped by the weather into weird outcrops, hollowed overhangs, giant boulders, proud cliffs. On this particular day, we'd climbed a scrubby ridge to some cliffs, and came to a point where we had to traverse a cliffy section, crossing midway over a deep but narrow cleft in the rock. A woman called Kate took the lead. She'd done this before, and climbed skilfully across with her backpack. Then she coaxed us over one by one, taking our packs from us as we stepped over the cleft.

She was the person I would have been, before my fall at Ndala. She was strong and funny, she even shared my name. Kate #1 had to ask one of the guys to hand my pack to her, because I couldn't do it. Then she talked me across as you would a scared child. I felt sick. My legs shook. The drop below made me dizzy. I was Kate #2 now.

In time, Kate #2 regained some of her courage. She took up rock climbing with a new boyfriend not that long after. But she wasn't quite the same, was she?

Cut back to the present, where I've taken another fall. Life is showing me yet again that I can't take it for granted.

11 September

Pain is a ruthless teacher. I had any number of accidents in my youth, but never hurt myself badly. I fell out of trees, got tossed off my horse, crashed my bicycle, sat on ant nests, and no doubt learnt a measure of caution from each. But my fall at Ndala Gorge was my first experience of severe pain.

Afterwards, no matter what my mind thought about the whole process, my body took over and instructed me to watch myself. Don't be cocky, take it easy, climb carefully. In the Grampians, my body delivered up a milder version of previous events: nausea, shaking, fear. Making sure I didn't forget the consequences of my rashness. How wonderful that I can look after myself so.

Which is why my experience of cancer has been so bewildering. The lump in my breast caused me no pain. And if the cancer had spread to other parts of my body, the new lumps wouldn't have hurt either. Not until they grew big enough to make other things hurt.

Before Cancer Day, I was in great shape. Despite being old enough to have teenage daughters, I was slim, active, apparently healthy. I avoided preservatives, chemicals, plastic food containers – I even put on daggy reading glasses in supermarkets so I could check food labels. I cooked with good ingredients and ate plenty of fruit and vegetables. And nor was I a fanatic – even that I'd thought through. Self-deprivation and obsessive food management create stress, and we all know stress is bad, bad, bad. Moderation is best, that was my motto.

I went into surgery feeling sad but well, and woke up with my world in disarray. Now I was in pain, but the pain was good for me. That's what I was meant to believe. My tumour was gone, yay! Along with all the lymph nodes in my armpit and a good chunk of my right boob. Blood-tinged lymphatic fluid drained from a tube under my arm, and another tube drained my breast. A cannula emptied saline solution and painkillers from an IV bag into the back of my hand.

The muscles across my back and shoulder ached, my underarm was numb. I couldn't lie comfortably on my right side for months. The drain tube under my arm stayed in for two weeks as my lymphatic system tried to rebuild itself. I could feel the embedded tube as a niggling pain when I moved. After a week, undrained fluid built up in my armpit and I had to have it aspirated (sucked out with a needle). Then the drain entry wound got infected – more drugs for me. I was still taking antibiotics when I started chemo.

What a way to crash. But I'm supposed to celebrate the pain.

12 September

I'm fascinated by the idea of people's energy fields – those lifelines that surround us all, radiating the flow of energy within.

When my kids were little, I practised trying to see auras, but never knew if the odd blotches of colour I saw were simply eye strain from staring in one spot too long. And eventually I decided what's the point anyway – do I really want or need to know what's going on with people? Because that's what it's about, isn't it? Having insider knowledge about someone's emotional/mental state?

Anyway around that time I read that younger kids can often see auras, so I questioned my daughter, who was maybe four or five at the time. Something along the lines of 'When you look at people, do you ever see colours?'

'Yeah.'

'Where do you see them?'

She put the flat of her hand about three centimetres above my wrist and said, 'There. The colours are all around you.'

Well, that got me going, didn't it! I asked about some of the people we knew, and for each she rattled off a list of colours. I think mine were pink, blue, purple, orange and gold. I asked her what she thought the colours meant, and that too she could tell me.

'Pink is relaxed, blue is frustrated, purple is noisy/loud, red is angry, white is cold (snow), green is relaxed, orange is the sun, yellow is hot (nice hot), gold is happy, grey is sad/crying/pain, black is dark (night).'

Even our dog (a mopey whippet) had labels: pink and green (when relaxed), purple (when barking), grey (when sad, left behind).

I didn't want to make a big deal about what she was seeing in case she told others and they laughed at her. But every now and then I'd ask if she could see her special colours, and she'd nod yes. Then a few years later she looked at me as if I was crazy and asked what I was talking about.

Lately I've been thinking about auras again, not because I want to 'read' other people, but so I can read myself. Has my thinking and analysing – the constant patter in my head – been obscuring from me some home truths? If I'd seen the signs, would I have fixed my life sooner? If I'd been happier with myself earlier, would I have avoided cancer?

Blue should be my colour for today.

I've tried a few times and still can't see my aura, so I've developed a revised technique. It's simple – I just visualise my body and observe what colours come to mind.

Here goes. Relaxing, breathing slowly…

Murkiness, yep lots of that. A thick sludginess in my upper legs, and over my right breast a burst of red with the outer edge sliced flat. The hump on my back, the one I mentioned earlier, is dark green, brown, weighty. I see shards of electric blue in my upper body. And my head? Grey/white like my hair, now dyed platinum blonde to hide the grey.

Well, go figure. That's not sounding good.

13 September

It's Mum's birthday. She's eighty-six. Happy birthday, Mum. I'm sorry for all the grief I've caused you. Not so much right now – these days she's less shocked by the crap life tosses her way – no, I'm thinking about the sleepless nights she had years ago, waiting for my car lights to appear in the driveway in the early hours of the morning after a party in the city. Or her waving me off on my bushwalking escapades in my little car – a rusty old bomb with sagging suspension, playing chicken on the highways with semi-trailers. Or when I hoisted my pack and flew off to India by myself, and only rang home three times in as many months.

Did I tell her about the time I almost toppled over a cliff in the Flinders Ranges when I sidestepped a bush and the weight of my pack tipped me towards the edge? Or when I drove our old Landrover to the very brink of the bank overlooking our dam and then couldn't get it into reverse? (Another centimetre forward, that's all it needed…) Or when I sat on top of the cabin of a large truck in India as we careered down a switchback road in the mountains, watching the littered carcasses of fallen trucks far below?

I didn't tell her any of that. But it's her birthday, let's celebrate the good.

My mum is a quiet achiever. She doesn't reveal what she's thinking very often, but when she does it's astonishing how spot on she is. She's a storyteller, and loves to speak of her childhood and younger years. It was a different era back then, and she connects me to a world that was more innocent and less informed – perhaps in a better way. A time when you dealt with the immediate world around you, and the rest didn't (couldn't) matter. We know too much these days, don't we?

Mum's creative. Her flower arrangements are unusual and often inspired. Even in a house full of kids and pets, dirty washing and an endless list of chores waiting to be done, she always had flowers on display. She still does.

She paints simple but striking landscapes, and any craft you can think of she's tried. I have many of her gifts: paintings; needlework cushion covers, pictures and bookmarks; home-made cards; a knitted jumper she made for me in my early twenties; a stained-glass star; a hand-painted wooden key ring holder cut in the shape of a cow.

I don't think life panned out the way she hoped it would, but she made do. She raised nine kids – and what an undertaking that was – without ever complaining, even though she once admitted she would happily have stopped at four. But if she'd done that, I wouldn't exist.

Thanks, Mum, I love you.

14 September

Speaking of road trips in old cars reminds me of an occasion when it wasn't me behind the wheel. I can't remember why my brother Michael decided to take his car; maybe I talked him into it. I hope not. Back then, he had a Dodge Phoenix that was his pride and joy. It was brave of him, owning a car like that, since most of his peers owned hotted-up Holden Monaros and other rev-head mobiles.

The Phoenix was spectacular. It had a bonnet stretching from here to eternity, and a wondrous push-button gear change that spoke of life in the slow lane. This car was a cruiser, low-throated and low-slung. And it had bucketloads of room, with a boot that swallowed our bulky packs, and legroom fit for royalty.

I sat beside Mike and we hit the highway.

Not far out of the city, on a stretch notorious for trucks, we got stuck behind a slow car. Everyone was busy talking and paid little attention as Mike drummed his fingers on the wheel and peered into the distance, waiting for his chance.

At the first break in the traffic, he accelerated, then pulled back again as he worked out his fully loaded car needed more space. I stopped talking and started watching. Then came another break and he gunned it, the big car pulling into the right lane with ease. But the car in front seemed to be speeding up, and the shimmering tarmac ahead was no longer empty. A semi-trailer was barrelling towards us.

Just as Mike floored it, I gasped and told him not to overtake. He hesitated, braking, then I realised the car beside us was braking too.

'Go faster!' I yelled through the deadly silence in the cabin.

He gunned it again, but now the truck was close.

'I won't make it,' he shouted, and I don't know what I said but I'm sure it was unhelpful.

Mike slammed on the brakes and swung the car off the road to the right, kicking gravel in the path of the semi as it roared past. Grit sprayed over his car's shining duco as he pulled to a stop.

We sat in stunned silence, dust billowing around us.

If I'd kept my trap shut, we would have been fine. I knew, absolutely, that I could have killed us all.

And that wasn't the end of it. I won't even start on how Mike took his beautiful car along the bumpy tracks to where we started our bushwalk, banging the low sump on rocks and scraping the paintwork on prickly acacias. And how on the return trip the car broke down on a deserted road, forcing us to walk kilometres for help and extending our trip by two days.

More rocks.

15 September

I'm back in the café of the hospital where I got radiation therapy, which could be seen as a step back or a rousing step forward. I'm picking the latter, or attempting to. Time to remind myself of what I've been through, and what it's all for.

I came to this hospital thirty times to be zapped. Thirty times I got up, showered, dressed and wrapped my bald head in a scarf – ready to strip off and bare my damaged chest to a bunch of technicians.

Here's the routine. Drive twenty-five minutes to the hospital, walk to the radiation oncology section, scan my treatment card at the main desk, proceed to the patients' waiting room, pick up a basket and hospital gown, smile at the people waiting their turn, go into a cubicle, change into my creased baby blue gown, then sit down in the stuffy waiting room with my basket full of clothes and valuables beside me.

Then came the waiting. This could be a few minutes or an hour depending on the status of the radiotherapy machines, which were frequently breaking down or being serviced. I often had time to chat with the regulars while flipping through trashy magazines, eyeing off the baskets of home-knitted beanies for baldies, and surreptitiously studying other patients to work out what was wrong with them.

Older men with bare legs and socks, their shirts showing under their blue gowns? Prostate. Women wearing pants and shoes, their top half bare under their gowns? Breast cancer most likely. Women without pants or skirts? Uterine or cervical cancer perhaps, or any range of abdominal cancers. Fully clothed people with no hair? Brain or skin cancer. Older people usually had hair, younger people not. There weren't many younger people there, and the ones I remember were women. Breast cancer, most of them.

There's a whole world of cancer out there, in every part of the body. I'm just guessing what people had; what would I know? I didn't ask them. They volunteered if they felt like it. I wanted to know of course. Who doesn't?

Who'd have thought this hospital microcosm existed with four linear accelerators running nine hours a day, nine days a fortnight, treating thirty patients each per day? That's around 120 people at any one time in my town getting radiotherapy.

Linear accelerators, or Linacs for those in the know, are the suns in the radiation oncology solar system. Four impressive pieces of technology housed in separate wings – each with medics shuttling in and out bringing offerings of sick patients.

Before my first treatment, I was introduced to the staff of LA 2, which was to be 'my' machine, but over the seven weeks I was treated by all four machines. Each LA featured a large rotating arm which could zap any part of the body as required. The ceiling above each treatment bed featured a pretty floral scene, and staff supplied music to pacify the sickies. As far as these things go, the rooms were quite pleasant.

When it was my turn to be zapped, a technician ushered me to the one of the LA rooms and directed me to a bench, where I deposited my basket of clothes, removed my gown and wrapped a clean sheet around myself. Then over to the machine where I lay as instructed on my back on the ineptly named 'bed'. They asked me to put my arms behind my head and discreetly slipped the sheet off my chest. Once I'd supplied my full name, age and address, we indulged in a few lines of polite conversation, then the two technicians got down to business.

I lay pretending I was elsewhere as they aimed red laser beams at my chest and marked my skin with black texta. As they worked, they read out numbers to each other, double-checking my position, and if either was dissatisfied, they continued moving the bed in tiny increments until both were happy. Precise positioning was crucial: the exact same area had to be irradiated each time. This is what took the time – the actual zapping took seconds.

Once strapped in place (I'm kidding), I was told not to move while the technicians hightailed it out of the room. In my case, they never shut the massive, concrete-filled doors behind them, but for some patients they had to (not kidding). As they huddled in the viewing cubicle with its big red button labelled NUKE! (kidding again), all I had to do was lie motionless and wait. Soon the warning lights came on and LA 1,2,3 or 4 beamed me with X-rays: generally fifteen to sixteen seconds from the right side, thirteen to fourteen from the left. I counted many times.

Then lights on, dismount, re-robe, say goodbye, walk out, get dressed, visit a nurse or doctor if an allotted day, scan card at front desk and…home.

Repeat twenty-nine times.

Simple? At first, yes.

Radiotherapy works in a similar way to chemotherapy. It targets the body's most active cells – cancer cells in particular – and damages or kills them. While normal cells often recover, cancer cells do not. In my case, the target zone was my right breast, which had been carefully tattooed with three grey dots to allow exact positioning of the beam during treatment.

Despite the indignity of being stretched out day after day on a hard bed with laser beams tracing across my scarred and tattooed chest, for a while it felt as if nothing was happening. I'd go home with texta marks on my skin and a sore spine (I had no padding after my rounds of chemo), feeling a little tired but pleased that I was withstanding things so well.

Skin cells take a hit from radiation because they're so active, and after three to four weeks, my skin started pinking up (in a perfect square over my breast and underarm). I continued diligently rubbing cream on each day and by the end my skin was red and sore, but tolerable.

Then the fatigue kicked in. Not sleepy tiredness, something worse. My muscles and joints stiffened up, and my fingertips started to tingle and sometimes go numb. Nearing the end of my treatment, I knew what it was like to be old: everything creaked and groaned, and my muscles hurt after the slightest activity. By the end, there was only one way to explain it: I felt like I'd been run over by a truck.

The side effects of radio are delayed and cumulative. My cells continued floundering and dying for a couple of weeks after treatment, and then they had to start the process of healing. It was over two months before I felt even half normal.

Unbelievably, nearly a year later I can still feel the effects.

But, and it's a big one – if there were any cancer cells left in my breast after surgery and chemo, then radiotherapy sounded their death knell. Girl, keep your eye on the ball.

16 September

Silly me thinking that hanging out in the hospital café yesterday would help somehow. I didn't even need to go there. But I'd developed a taste for the café's ham and cheese croissants so it seemed a good plan: get breakfast while I was down that way, and take some time to reflect.

Bah humbug. The croissants were greasy and unpleasant; I hope I never eat them again. And being at the hospital reminded me of the helplessness I felt while undergoing treatment. Other people had control over my body, and my mental state was immaterial.

Cancer Kate. That's me.

Until recently, I considered myself to be fairly solid, underneath it all, but now I don't feel that. At my centre is squishy marshmallow.

What to do, what to do?

Perhaps there's something in my recurring theme of rocks. Rocks = heaviness, but also strength. Solidity. Give me a rocky outcrop to sit on, or the top of a cliff, or a jumble of boulders by the ocean and my spirits lift.

Maybe what I need is a café selling decent ham and cheese croissants on top of a cliff.

*

I've been reading a book about intuition. The idea that our energy is connected, that none of us are truly separate. We all have access to a greater knowledge – not just within ourselves but from the energy of the universe. I guess it's like connecting with our soul, or our spiritual guides or however you want to see it.

You can scoff if you like, but given my current state of mind I'm keeping my options open.

So earlier today I found myself a quiet spot to lie down and tune in to my intuition. My mind was buzzy and for a while all I got was mind chatter. Then a memory came to me.

It's hot. I've come up from the city to visit my parents, and I'm out for a walk in the orchard. The road I'm walking on has been graded recently so there's a layer of powdery dirt in the ruts. As I approach the spray shed, I see my brother Michael next to one of our tractors. He waves and walks down to join me, still holding a heavy tractor chain.

We stand on the dirt track, chatting. He swings the chain idly, I kick at the ground with my sandshoe sending puffs of dust into the air.

Maybe he looks a little glum, or maybe it's just sisterly chat but I ask him, 'Are you happy, Mike?'

He says yes.

That's all I remember from the conversation. I kept on with my walk and he went back to the tractor. It was the last time I saw him.

Did he know, then? And why didn't I know? Where was my intuition on that day?

But this wasn't meant to be a self-flagellation exercise. I shook these thoughts away and tried to relax. Finally I felt suitably calm, ready to ask my intuition (or my higher self, whatever) what I needed to know.

The answer took a while and was a bit weak, but what I got was pretty simple: 'It's not that bad.' Yep, that was it. I worry too much.

What a let-down. Where was my blinding revelation, the get out of jail free card I was hoping for?

But no. *I worry too much.*

It was true of course, but what was I supposed to do about it? Stop worrying? Easier said than done.

After a while, my thoughts went back to that scene with Michael and replayed it. But this time as he stood there with me on the road I asked him for advice. He smiled at me and I felt his warmth. Then he let the tractor chain collapse onto the dirt and a tingling wave of release surged through me. Yes, he said, you do worry too much.

17 September

I read last night that if cancer moves from the breast and invades other parts of the body, it can't be cured – just contained. Managed. This scared the crap out of me.

What am I doing being so complacent? Waking every day to my sad breast and sad, sad soul – that should be enough of a reminder, shouldn't it? Seize the day, learn from my mistakes, be positive.

I'm tired of that mantra. Can I really avoid cancer by being more positive? My analytical brain keeps telling me it's just not that simple. Dogs get cancer. Mice can be genetically engineered to get cancer. Nobody blames the dogs and mice for their state of mind. Cancer is part of the great, complicated wheel of life.

So where does that leave me?

I was trained as a scientist, and I like to find neat solutions to things. Here's a biological theory for why I may have ended up with cancer.

The first clue was in my early twenties. I found a benign lump in my left breast, and was told that my breast tissue was 'granular' in texture (dense). (There's a ranking used in mammograms for breast density. Mine are rated as BI-RADS type 3 – heterogenously dense – in a scale from 1, least dense, to 4, most dense. This means I have more glandular – milk-producing – tissue than is necessary.) While this is fairly common, it's not ideal – but I didn't know that then. Only recently I learned that women with granular breasts are more prone to breast cancer and a history of benign lumps may also be a risk factor.

The second clue was a few years ago. I discovered I had an iron deficiency which had been worsening for years. Although taking iron corrected the problem, whenever I stopped, my iron levels began to fall. After a series of tests revealed nothing, I was told uterine fibroids could be the culprit as they cause heavy periods (blood loss = iron loss). Since fibroids are relatively benign, I didn't bother finding out if I had them – I figured all I had to do was keep taking iron until menopause and leave it at that. I didn't know fibroids can be caused by high oestrogen levels, and if I had, I wouldn't have worried. What's wrong with oestrogen? It's just a normal female hormone which regulates our reproductive processes.

Then I got cancer. And the CT scans I had after my diagnosis revealed – you guessed it – uterine fibroids. Too late, she cried.

What these clues add up to is oestrogen dominance. A big name for something simple – high oestrogen levels. And long-term exposure to oestrogen is a known risk factor for breast cancer. That vital hormone that allows us to be wondrously female and bring forth children into the world can be a devil in disguise.

Ironically, my cancer treatment has solved the iron problem. No more periods, no more blood loss. Easy. And my chemo-induced menopause (chemopause ☺) is lowering my blood oestrogen levels. Along with that, I'm now taking a drug to block the action of oestrogen in my body. So my oestrogen troubles should be over.

But what caused the high oestrogen levels in the first place?

Here's where I diverge into more alarming territory. Breast cancer is becoming more common. Girls are getting their periods earlier and generally have larger breasts. Why?

Our modern environment is full of chemicals which mimic the

action of oestrogen. We put these xenoestrogens on our skin (phthalates, parabens and other chemicals in cosmetics and toiletries) or absorb them from food or our environment (plastics, flame retardants, pesticides, herbicides and more). Is it possible that these chemicals, which contaminate women's breast tissue and breast milk the world over, are stimulating our bodies in the same way oestrogen does? Causing a kind of oestrogen overload syndrome? Add to this the synthetic oestrogens we ingest: the contraceptive pill and hormone replacement therapy, and the hormones in various animal products. Are these creating an oestrogenic time bomb in our bodies?

And there's more. Many women in our modern world have fewer pregnancies and babies, breastfeed for less time, get their periods earlier and start menopause later. This means they are exposed to oestrogen from a younger age and more regularly throughout their reproductive lives. Furthermore, they tend to start their families later in life, and having babies when younger is known to protect breast tissue from cancer.

All of this adds up to one big hormonal mess for women. And me. Or does it?

I've been avoiding nasty chemicals for years. I try not to store foods in plastic, especially fatty or hot foods. I've never owned a new car – I can't handle the smell, let alone the price. I don't use cleaning chemicals, I keep my home well-aired, I avoid chemicals in cosmetics and toiletries…the list goes on.

And as I've already pointed out, I haven't done too badly in the hormonal stakes, having avoided the pill (mostly), been pregnant before thirty (just) and breastfed both of my children. Nonetheless, I was showing signs of oestrogen dominance in my twenties. Why?

Perhaps I'm genetically predisposed to having high oestrogen levels. Or I'm particularly sensitive to those oestrogen-mimicking chemicals (xenoestrogens) which I suspect are so widespread that my efforts to avoid them are pointless.

It's also possible that emotions are indeed part of the equation –

since all women know how closely entwined emotions and hormones are. But has my emotional state over my lifetime been any different to most people's? Have I really been more stressed, more unhappy (less positive), more screwed up by life than anyone else?

Which brings me back to a state of confusion.

18 September

Today I'm wondering where I'm going with all of this. Is this meandering journey backwards and forwards through my life helping me? Do I feel any better? Are my spirits lifting? No. Each day still dawns with a slightly sad awakening. I have bright moments but not many. Mostly I'm overwhelmed, lost in a labyrinth.

It seems I hoped that pouring my heart out on the page would do something, open up something new and uplifting. Not yet.

I should stop pretending that I haven't taken a huge hit. When my oncologist said, 'We're going for gold,' his meaning was stark. I win by staying alive. Happiness isn't part of the equation.

*

There are ongoing effects from my cancer that I never thought of. I can no longer claim to be someone with an excellent health record. Travel insurance is harder to get. Life insurance is much harder.

And what about travelling to far-flung places? I've often thought about wangling a stint in Antarctica. Not just cruising in and out on a big tourist ship – although that would do for starters. I want to live there, work there. Experience it all. The ever-changing light, the myriad of weather moods the frozen continent is known for. I want to hear glaciers creaking and the roar of ice towers crashing into the sea. I want to go on research expeditions and see giant colonies of seabirds and penguins. Spend the night in a flimsy tent with the alien sounds of a frozen landscape around me. And I want to be trapped in an Antarctic base station as a blizzard rages outside.

If I could go there, I'd find a way to write about it without all these clichés.

But now cancer is stamped on my forehead. This is my lot. Even though my chances of recurrence are low. Even though I'm returning to my naturally robust state (yes, today I believe I am).

Sigh.

But just for today, I'm imagining this.

Lying on my narrow bunk, I listen to the steady throb of engines. The ocean is calmer now, and I can hear the scraping and dragging of ice against the ship's hull. I'm over my seasickness and feel strangely buoyant. The icebergs are outside now – my soul is clear.

Soon I'll stand on the ice. Me, Kate.

It's not much of an adventure in the scheme of things. I've come here in relative luxury. I won't be trekking across the ice with my sledge and dogs heading for the South Pole. Other people are stronger than I'll ever be. But this place is magic, and I made it here. If the world has a consciousness, then surely this is the centre.

Of course the cold will be unbelievable, the research centre full of stir-crazy people and I'll be calling home in no time. But still.

19 September

Yesterday in the supermarket I turned into aisle 4 and did a double take. A magpie was staring down at me from its perch on a box of washing powder. As I wheeled my trolley closer, it glanced up at the fluorescent lights, checking to see if blue sky had magically appeared, then flew across to the next aisle.

A staff person came around the corner and I asked her if she'd seen the bird.

'Sure,' she said. 'It's been here for a while. We can't get it out.'

It looked so out of place. Which got me thinking. Why was it sad for a bird to be trapped in such an unnatural environment but not me? I chose to come into this supermarket with its over-bright artificial light, shiny floors and shelves stacked with products cloaked in plastic, cardboard, glass, metal. I was breathing in recycled air loaded with chemical gases, I was buying foods wrapped in petrochemicals, I was walking on the unnaturally flat floor in shoes that distanced not just my feet but my whole body from the earth.

Yes, it got me thinking.

And today looking around my office, what can I see that comes direct from nature? There are a few seashells on the top shelf of my bookcase, a daddy longlegs spider above the door and there's me and the dog. That's it. Everything else is artificial: manufactured or altered in one way or another.

Who am I kidding? Worrying that my cancer is a result of my (faulty) state of mind when there are clues all around me? Thinking that I'm more stressed or emotionally dysfunctional than everyone else?

And who are we kidding thinking that somehow we are more burdened by life's concerns than the generations proceeding us? Two hundred years ago, I'd be terrified of dying in labour, or of my children dying of any number of infectious diseases. I'd be working my fingers to the bone washing clothes by hand, carting wood for fires, growing food and watching it being ruined by drought or flood, hail or fire. You think that's not stressful?

My guess is that humans are pretty well adapted for stress. All animals must be, surely. Look at my dog Chico. He lives a fabulous life compared to his wild counterparts, but does he know for sure when his next meal will arrive? Nope. Every afternoon his anxiety starts to mount as he waits and hopes. His worried eyes follow me around and his little brain whirrs. 'Will she feed me? Oh, please let her feed me.'

Then finally as I carry his loaded bowl outside, he bounces around me with waggy tail and bright eyes, doing his little doggy dance. He can't believe his luck. Once more, the human has done her job.

And what about the rabbits that he likes to chase in the bush near our house? Do you think they sit outside their burrows chatting and enjoying the sunshine? Oh no, every instant they're on alert, looking, smelling, preparing. 'Look! A human and a dog!' Run rabbit run (hop, whatever).

*

Like a rabbit, my thoughts are running round and round.

I'm reminded of a time several years ago when I mistakenly believed stress to be making me unwell.

My girls were younger, my husband was often overseas, and I kept things going at home without much help. Life was full-on, so it was easy to explain the range of minor ailments I began noticing as due to lack of sleep, anxiety, poor eating, too much booze – nothing unusual there.

But my symptoms began to pile up and I started wondering what the hell was wrong with me. I was tired and sleeping badly, often jerking awake feeling like I was suffocating or with my heart jumping. Some nights, I bit my cheek or tongue and woke up with blood in my mouth. During the day, my heartbeat was irregular and I found myself puffing when hardly doing anything. People kept telling me I was pale and wan.

My response was to chastise myself for getting overstressed. I needed to take time out, to meditate, walk, be nice to myself. Drink less, eat better, be more assertive, be more positive…yah de yah and on it went.

Then one awful, awful day I had a seizure. The first I knew of it was when I came to with an ambulance person beside me. I was carted off to hospital and given all the tests, but no cause was established. Maybe it was a one-off, maybe it was the beginnings of epilepsy. All I could do was wait and see.

So I got super-healthy, gave up alcohol, exercised more and tried to get my head around what had happened. The months ticked by with no more seizures, and for a while I felt a bit better. Then I lapsed into more usual behaviour – rushing around, trying to do everything at once, exercising less, drinking alcohol, eating more haphazardly – and my symptoms got worse again. I knew I should be careful but honestly thought after so long another seizure was unlikely.

Wrong. After the second seizure, I really took a hit. This time, my symptoms didn't subside. Once again I wasn't driving, and I was told if I had more seizures I should go on epilepsy medication. This terrified me – I didn't want drugs that messed with my mind.

So I started doing more research, and noticed that both sets of blood tests from after my seizures revealed slightly low blood haemoglobin levels. Not enough for my GP to think it warranted investigation (even though one report recommended further iron studies) and the results were pushed aside.

When I did some reading about haemoglobin and the symptoms of iron deficiency, I was shocked. All of my symptoms (except the seizures) were a match. I rushed out and got some iron tablets. Within days my symptoms started to go. And when I got a blood test my suspicions were confirmed – abnormally low iron levels, probably developed over years.

In the next few months, I kept taking iron and all of those niggling symptoms disappeared. I haven't had a seizure since.

Doctors don't seem to like my suggestion that iron deficiency could have given me seizures, but five years on I'm pretty convinced. Iron allows your blood cells to carry oxygen around the body. Every organ is affected by lack of oxygen, including the heart and brain. Important neurotransmitters need iron. So for someone with a susceptible brain (I knew I was a bit whacko), it's plausible, I reckon.

But back to my main point. I fluffed around for months – no, years – telling myself that if I could just manage my stress levels I'd start feeling better. At some point, my husband suggested I take iron pills but I ignored him. I'd tried various supplements over the years and they didn't agree with my digestive system. They weren't for me. What I needed was to fix up my mind.

Wrong. All I needed was iron.

Okay, it's not quite that simple, since my iron troubles turned out to be linked to other things – but it's interesting, isn't it?

22 September

All right, it's time to fess up. Of the known risk factors for breast cancer, there's a teensy little one I've been skirting around.

Alcohol.

Most women who've had children will appreciate the guilt load that comes with drinking. At the end of a long day, with the kiddlies finally (OMG, finally) in bed – who hasn't reached for a bottle of wine? Not every night, oh no. And mostly just one glass, even if it is full to the brim. Then again some nights call for two, and as for nights with the girls, well hey – let's crack open another champers.

Now it seems my one vice, my one guilty pleasure, is trouble. Even light drinking – one measly standard drink a day – can raise the risk of breast cancer.

Noooo!

I'm not stupid – I know alcohol ain't good for me – so even when I was drinking regularly, I made an effort to abstain for at least three nights a week, two of them in a row. I think that's reasonable. Like everything, it's not simple. If alcohol were such a high risk, every second woman would have breast cancer. (Unless it's the guilt that comes with drinking that's the risk factor? Just a thought. Okay, scratch that one.)

For the moment, I'm not drinking much at all, but in the future I don't know. Isn't there a benefit to putting your feet up at the end of day with a nice sauvignon blanc in hand? That moment where you go 'Ah…life's good' – isn't there value in that?

23 September

When people explained what to expect during my treatment, they took time to walk me through the details. They seemed thorough. And they were – given the limitations of time and money, and the unpredictability of the human body. Because, as it turned out, there was plenty I wasn't warned about. Like my arms. Both of them ended up as casualties – who'd have thought?

It started with surgery. A flow-on effect from having the lymph nodes removed from my underarm was some kind of stress damage to the lymphatic vessels in my right arm. Cording, it was called, when I finally found someone who could tell me what was going on. The connective tissue around the lymph vessels was scarred, making the vessels less flexible. They pulled tight like cords when I lifted my arm.

After surgery, I avoided lifting my arm very high (given the wounds on my chest and underarm) but when I finally got around to doing the exercises I'd been given, my right arm wouldn't lift much above half-mast. OMG.

Diligently I kept up the exercises and slowly my arm started to free up. But by then I'd started chemotherapy, and I noticed my left forearm getting a bit sore from the exercises. I put it down to lack of activity, but after the third round of chemo, it was clear what was going on.

The epirubicin, as I knew, was burning my veins when injected through my IV line. But what I hadn't considered was that every round of chemo was searing another vein, and exacerbating the damage to the veins used in the previous rounds. By the fourth round of chemo, my left arm couldn't straighten properly and the back of my wrist and hand ached constantly. Sunken purple veins became visible, running from my hand to above my forearm. I could feel them like sore ropes in my armpit.

When I went for my final round of chemo, my veins were so scarred and damaged it took them twenty minutes to get the cannula in. Lucky I'd taken Ativan to help me chill or I'd have passed out.

For weeks afterwards, my forearm was a horror show of hard, purple veins. I carried my left arm tucked into my side because otherwise it hung awkwardly, bent and hurting, unable to straighten. I called it the 'Claw'.

Five months later, I can straighten my arm but the misshapen veins remain. Still sunken, still hard. Freakish. As for my right arm, it aches when I carry heavy bags, and gets sore from tiny amounts of house work. My underarm is numb and sore to touch. If I don't do my exercises, everything starts to seize up again.

So I'm left with two dysfunctional arms as well as a sore underarm and breast.

If I had to put a name to what I've found hardest about my cancer, it wouldn't be fear. Or pain. Not even sadness. It'd be loss.

24 September

A visitor this morning told me that our house makes him feel calm. I said it's because of me, then laughed and said actually I'm often not calm at all. But in truth the way our house feels has a lot to do with me. I go to a lot of effort to make wherever I live look nice. Feel nice. People often comment on that.

I'm starting to think I do this because I'm thin-skinned. I soak up the moods, the feeling of situations, people, places. Some would say my boundaries are fuzzy, and that's most likely true. When I'm with people, that can be a problem, but in nature it's mostly good. Like right now when I look out my bedroom window at the wattle bush heavy with golden flowers, and laugh at the Indian mynah hanging upside-down from a branch enjoying a feed. The big gum tree across the road shakes in the wind, while the recently pruned diosma bush right outside the window ripples gently.

In my home, almost every window has a view of bushes and garden. Each glance outside, however brief, gives me a tiny lift. The energy of nature seeps through me. I need that right now, more than ever.

25 September

Yesterday I saw my surgeon: just a routine visit to see how I'm going. A physical examination, a bit of a chat to make sure I have no suspicious symptoms. And so far, so good; I appear to be fine. Was I worried before I went? I don't think I was.

I can't work this out: why have I been so unconcerned? Most women say they're terrified once their treatment ends. Every twinge, every odd feeling has them freaking out.

Have I been hiding from my fear? Sticking my head in the sand and waiting for it all to go away?

Before all this, I believed my life would work out all right, one way or another. Why? After all, my nephew died, and my brother – there's nothing all right about that. My sister lost her child and her brother.

My parents lost their grandson, then their son, and finally the family business in the space of ten years. Sometimes it hurt me more seeing their pain than feeling my own.

And yet despite all that, I managed to keep hoping. Believing in a rosy future. Is that what everyone does when they're young? Is it that simple?

Either which way, now the hope is draining away.

Which brings me back to loss. I'm grieving, that's what's going on. Grieving for the loss of my youth, my foolish optimism, my 'she'll be right, mate' attitude. Aiee.

There's a lot going on in my life right now. Work stuff, family stuff, me stuff. Like a sponge, I'm soaking up emotions from all directions and they're clogging me up.

Going down, going down…

Earlier today I lay on my bed and tuned into my energy. The rocks are still there, on my shoulders. My aura, my colours are so depleted I can hardly sense them. No wonder I'm not coping. No wonder I feel like a sponge – the forcefield I need to keep me safe is full of holes.

There's an exercise I learnt once from a massage therapist who also worked on energy healing. She told me to stand barefoot, outside if possible, and visualise breathing in the energy of the earth from my feet right through to my head, then breathing it out the top of my head into the sky. Next she said breathe in the energy of the heavens (sun, wind, rain, stars!) and draw it down through my body to my feet then into the earth like a river of energy.

When I do this now, I feel the energy rattling through me like the wind blowing autumn leaves along the gutters.

27 September

Yesterday I cut my toenails and I'm nearly there – only a millimetre of mutant nails to go. Next time, I'll be able to remove all traces of my chemo. It's like looking at the stars and seeing the past in action – watching my scarred, misshapen nails slowly progressing up my nail bed, reminding me of the supernova once lived through.

All right, it's five a.m. and I'm getting melodramatic. Wish I could go back to sleep.

There has to be – has to be – some good I can take away from all this.

6 October

Physically I'm on the mend. It's three months since I finished radiotherapy and I've got some of my strength back. While I'm not fit like I was, that's easily remedied. My underarm is a bit tight and numb but that may take years to go completely. My chemo arm looks bad but doesn't stop me doing everyday activities any more. My fingertips are still frequently numb, and it's really bugging me. But I reckon that'll pass soon.

Boring details. On the surface, I'm mostly okay now. And yet it's a façade. Do I feel okay? Nowhere near it.

Trouble is, my sympathy vote has run out. You can get away with talking about how bad you feel when you're obviously unwell. But now people tell me that I'm glowing. 'You look great! Your hair really suits you!' They don't want to hear that I'm not okay. That I'm dull and dreary and utterly BOGGED. They want me to move on.

Hmph.

This feeling I have isn't that different to how I felt when my brother died. When we die, we are so utterly alone. My brother sat himself against a tree looking over the city, and he died. Alone. For months after, when I lay in bed with my veil of grief around me, this unbearable truth kept me awake. Most of our lives we spend alone, even when we're with others. Luckily we're pretty good at evading this knowledge. I recovered from my grief; I threw myself back into busyness. No doubt I can do it again. But right now all I can feel is the loneliness like cold water lapping at my feet.

This isn't helping, right? Shaking it off, shaking it off...

9 October

My mistake, or one of them anyway, is in believing that others can fix my problems. I often offload my worries onto others – partly for reassurance and partly in the hope that the telling will free me. If I understand, I can let go, right?

It seems not. Talking about my issues often feels like a cheap fix. I feel better, temporarily, but what does it change?

I had some counselling during my cancer treatment. It was a free service, and I appreciated sitting with someone and talking without fear of blame and criticism. Counsellors are paid to say the right things and be supportive – we all know that – but nonetheless I did feel supported. I really liked the woman I saw, and in another life we could be friends. But the last time I went, I left feeling frustrated. Was all this talking helping me? Was it teaching me to go out in the world and really believe in myself?

Nope. In my usual manner, I'd been hoping she'd trigger some momentous event in my psyche enabling me to take hold of my life and make it better.

The ball's back in my court. Again.

Besides, when I need a listening ear, there's always my friends. They say the right things; they care about me. I walk away feeling better, even if no better equipped to deal with my life.

*

Several years ago, I tried a session of breathwork. It was soon after my first seizure when I was casting about, trying to find out what was going on. Breathwork didn't give me the answers, but it gave me plenty to think about. Most of all, it made me aware of the power of our hidden selves. No matter what our thinking minds let us believe, much of our behaviour is driven by that sleeping giant: our subconscious.

Sceptical?

Here's how it went for me. After a bit of a chat with the lovely woman guiding the session, I lay down on a couch and got comfy. The woman, who I'll call Cherie, asked me to take quick, shallow breaths. I didn't like this because it reminded me of the EEG scan I had after my first seizure, where they got me to hyperventilate in the hope it'd bring on another seizure. It was destabilising, a technique designed to put me on edge.

Finally, Cherie let me go back to normal breathing. As I lay there feeling shaky, she began asking me how I felt in certain situations when young. At first I spoke awkwardly, but then the weirdest thing happened. Powerful emotions began to fill me, like I was reliving them.

At one point I started crying about an incident when I was really young, where I was upset but my parents were distracted by my other siblings and pretty much ignored me. What amazed me (afterwards) was how my adult self watched over all this distantly, while this childish self spoke to Cherie about events as if I was still there, racked by the frustrations and hurts I felt as a child.

Afterwards I walked away feeling as if something momentous had happened. I'd tuned into my childhood self and relived some powerful emotions.

In breathwork, the thinking is that by exposing these negative emotional memories, we can release ourselves from them. So had I released the monsters?

No. I felt lighter in the same way I do after a good massage. But did it bring on any lasting changes in my emotional state? I can't say I noticed anything. I suppose it takes time. Maybe I should go back for more sessions. But I probably won't.

And here's a thought. If the lessons we learn during our childhood influence how we continue living our lives, then surely an early hurt can lead us through a chain of interconnected experiences and emotions leading right up to the present? To really be free, perhaps we have to work our way along the whole chain, releasing all the hurts and upsets all the way along.

That's sounding like hard work.

10 October

Negativity gets tiring. I'm so over it. It's easy to focus on the negatives in life, harder, much harder to hold onto the positives. But here's one.

Earlier this month, we stayed for three nights in a high-rise apartment complex right on the beach in northern NSW. From our balcony, we watched a procession of whales swimming past in little groups. Humpback whales with their young, returning to the cooler waters of Antarctica from breeding grounds further north.

Almost every time I went out onto the balcony, I'd spot some, coming to the surface with their spouts of water dissipating above them. Sometimes I could see a tail curving out and then down into the water again, sometimes a fin.

The breakers near the shore were littered with surfers avidly trying to stake their claim on the best waves. I wondered how many of them knew who they were sharing the ocean with. I don't know why but I found the presence of the whales comforting. Perhaps because it reminded me that not everything in life revolves around humans.

12 October

My aunty Rosemary died today. Another soul released into the next world, wherever that is. I found out through Facebook, of all places. That's the kind of world we live in now. No need for phone calls or death notices in newspapers any more.

My father has, or had, three younger sisters and now two of them are gone. Another reason why getting older sucks.

When I learnt that Rosemary had died, I sat for a while thinking about her. I hadn't seen much of her in years, so mostly I remember her from when she was younger. She was opinionated, funny, strong-willed. I remember her laughing a lot. If I visualise her now, she's with her sister Audrey, her mum Edna, her dad Alfred. And her daughter Anne, who wasn't a lot older than me when she died of cancer. Michael and Simeon are there too, taking off their motorbike helmets for a quick break in between rides.

These people who make up a part of my life only exist now in my memory, and that of the others who knew them. But they're not entirely gone. I feel them around me. I carry them with me.

13 October

I've been busier lately. It helps stave off the gloom, but only just. Where's my sunshine, my laughter? I have a growing conviction that this feeling is partly chemical. I think the hormone therapy drug I'm taking is messing with my moods – blocking the natural action of hormones already in tumult from my fast-tracked menopause.

It took three rounds of chemo to shunt me over the line – thirty-four years of periods stopped dead. And because my periods haven't returned, most likely that's it for me – I'm reproductively kaput. Another thing to grieve.

Because I have no experience of how normal menopause feels, I can't tell if my chemopause/hormonal therapy combo is any different. All I can say is that what I'm feeling isn't me. Even at my lowest ebbs, I've never felt like this.

If Tamoxifen – my hormonal therapy drug – is making me feel this way, then I've a problem. A big one. The effectiveness of modern breast cancer treatments is well established, and for cancers like mine hormonal therapy is an important part of the treatment. It significantly reduces the likelihood of cancer returning.

Most forms of breast cancer are what is known as hormonally receptive – which means they're stimulated by one or both of the hormones oestrogen and progesterone. My cancer is strongly hormonally receptive for both.

Tamoxifen is a clever little molecule that parks itself in the oestrogen receptors on cells all over the body. It means oestrogen molecules circulating in the body have less cells to bind to, including any nasty cancer cells waiting around for an oestrogen hit. In breast cells (including cancerous ones), Tamoxifen blocks the action of oestrogen. But in the bones and uterus Tamoxifen mimics the action of oestrogen while still blocking oestrogen itself. So in some ways Tamoxifen helps reduce the effects of menopause, just like HRT, while protecting the breast from that potential aggressor – oestrogen.

I'm meant to take it for around two years, then possibly switch to an aromatase inhibitor drug which is more effective in post-menopausal women. Rather than blocking the action of oestrogen, these drugs stop oestrogen production altogether. It's hard to imagine such drugs won't affect my moods too. Five years of feeling like this? It makes me shiver.

*

But I can't blame everything that's wrong with my life on Tamoxifen, and I'm not ready to stop taking it. On with the show.

14 October

I like the way small things can trigger a trail of thoughts spanning the past, the future, people, feelings, life, the universe and everything.

Yesterday I spotted a swamp wallaby in the bush reserve just up the road from our house. These wallabies are fairly common but I don't see them very often. This was the second I'd seen in two days, which is unusual. No doubt they're venturing down to the lower slopes of the mountain, unable to resist the lush spring grass that has overtaken the normally dry terrain.

There are grey kangaroos everywhere in the reserve and, while I love to watch them, I have a special fondness for wallabies. Maybe it's their long muscular tails, or their fluffy faces with round ears and small muzzles. They're shy, and when startled they hunch down low and go go go.

Seeing the wallaby reminded me of the time I saw my first (and only) yellow-footed rock wallaby in the wild. I was on one of my first walks with the university bushwalking club and couldn't believe my luck. Yellow-footed rock wallabies are a listed threatened species with a very limited range.

Our wallaby appeared when we were walking through a rocky gorge in inland South Australia. It was halfway up the steep side of the gorge, looking down on us. We barely had time to admire its yellow banded tail and multicoloured pelt before it bounded up the steep rock face and disappeared over the top. They're not called rock wallabies for nothing.

It made my day.

On those long ago bushwalks, I always had a camera with me, and I took some great photos. Not of the rock wallaby, she was way too fast, but of the rocky landscapes I loved. Intense blue skies framing burnt orange cliffs, ancient grass trees guarding the quiet edges of gorges…

By then, I'd been taking photos for years. When I was younger, I had one of those Polaroid cameras that pop out a blank image which develops like magic in your hand. I still have some of them, like the one of me with bucky teeth. And the one of Simeon, my nephew who died when only nine.

Simeon was six years younger than me, so he was like another brother. Of course he loved to come and play with his tribe of aunties and uncles, and because he was no threat to us (unlike siblings), we loved to have him around. He had golden hair and a sunny personality, and he was smart. He used to solve the chess problems in the newspaper, which impressed me no end. I didn't have the patience for chess.

I let him ride my horse Prince sometimes. He never rode far – Prince was prone to doing erratic things, and I don't think Simeon was terribly impressed by horses. He, like my brothers, was a motorbike fiend. The orchard around home was constantly abuzz with the din of two stroke engines. I used to sneer about them and complain when they zoomed past me and my ambling horse, but secretly I liked them too.

It bugs me, though, that my memories of Simeon are dim. Is the fuzziness just another complication of cancer treatment? I feel like the edge has been stripped from my memories, but how can I know what I've forgotten?

One thing I do remember clearly is being at his house after he died. I recall standing for ages watching his pet tortoise swimming around in its aquarium, feeling intensely sad that Morty lived on while Simeon did not. It made no sense to me.

I lingered in the doorway to his bedroom and dragged my eyes over his things. Toys tossed haphazardly around as kids do, on his bedside table the Lego helicopter he'd only just been given for his birthday. That made me cry. And his clothes, discarded, recently worn – unbearable reminders of a life cut short. There's no end to that kind of pain.

It's nice that his grave is next to Michael's. They were closest in age, and spent a lot of time together playing with Matchbox cars and generally lying low in case my older brothers spotted them and caused trouble. As Simeon got older, he started coming on holidays with us – making up numbers as one by one my older siblings stopped joining the holiday entourage. I remember one trip to Coffin Bay when we stayed in a caravan park. I got the spare bed in the caravan while Simeon, Mike and Marty slept in a tent outside. Dad used to snore so loudly the whole caravan rocked, and I remember lying in my bunk and listening enviously as the boys bounced around inside their tent, laughing into the wee hours of the morning.

I wish I got to see Simeon grow up.

15 October

Am I climbing up a cliff face, hold by hold, finding a way back to myself?

I did a lot of rock climbing in my twenties. It was something that suited my muscly build and natural flexibility. I wasn't the most daring of climbers – I preferred top roping, protected by a rope from above – and let others do the lead climbing. But nothing beats that feeling of hauling myself onto a ledge or clifftop and sitting there, tired but exhilarated, looking out over a beautiful landscape.

Climbing is tough on fingers and toes. The latter get jammed into cracks or held rigidly in an attempt to grip onto a tiny ridge of rock. And fingertips? Well, they get trashed. Apart from the physical difficulty of just holding on, fingertips get squashed and scraped raw by the harsh rock.

But why am I thinking of fingertips? Because they're another casualty of my treatment.

As I've already said, they started feeling a bit numb halfway through my radiotherapy, and got progressively worse. Then my fingers and hands started playing up too. When I told my radiologist, she said it was unlikely to be a treatment side effect. If it didn't resolve soon, she said I should get it checked out.

A week ago, I picked up the phone. My surgeon was away for a month. A breast care nurse thought it might be a neck problem. A chemo ward nurse said it could be a chemo side effect, and if so there was nothing I could do about it. I freaked and booked in to see my oncologist.

He reassured me that the numbness and tingling weren't a side effect of the chemo drugs I'd been given. (If I'd had other chemo drugs? Sure!) He said the problem was probably in my neck and sent me off for an MRI, 'just to be sure'. Sure of what? Then it hit me: he was checking I didn't have a tumour in my neck.

This played on my mind quite badly, as you can imagine.

The scan was okay, of course. Just a couple of slightly compressed discs in my neck, pushing into the spinal cavity and irritating the nerves. It's likely the chemo weakened my collagen (so my osteopath later said), and this in combination with months of inactivity and the muscular stresses of radiotherapy probably caused the problem.

This is better by far than having a tumour, but is debilitating nonetheless. When I sleep, I have to keep changing position to stop my fingers and hands from going numb. Sometimes my hands burn with pain and the only thing that helps (a bit) is to lie flat on my back with no pillow. Which I hate. So I'm tired. My hands are weak. Prolonged sitting is torture.

Now I sound like I'm whingeing – but it's so frustrating. I want to be better!

Are my hands and fingers telling me something? Some might say this a sign of some deeper turmoil… Nope, not this time.

But nonetheless, it's a physical reminder of my cancer load. Those months of fear and pain clamping my neck, my voice. Dependency and weakness smothering me. I feel the tightness of it in my throat, and the load of it on my shoulders and back.

These effects are indefinable. It may take me a long time to heal.

18 October

Today I snipped off the last signs of chemo damage from my toenails. I can't remember when I did the same with my fingernails but it was surely weeks and weeks ago. They must grow faster, which is interesting. If you think about it in evolutionary terms, we must be adapted for wearing down our fingernails faster than our toenails.

The chemo is still affecting my hair. It's lovely and thick, and no greyer than it was before all this, but as it grows longer it gets more and more unruly. It's actually curly! I still do a double take sometimes when I look in the mirror. Weird. People say it's only temporary. The hair follicles will recover and my hair (along with my life presumably) will go back to normal. That's the theory anyway.

19 October

My youngest daughter turned sixteen today. Happy birthday, darling – you are so perfect. My love for you stretches from the tropics to the cold zones and back again. I won't embarrass her by saying anything else. Just…wow. She makes me so proud.

And in three months or so, my oldest daughter turns eighteen. Sigh. But how lucky am I to have such smart, sassy girls? When I look at them, I know I must be doing okay as a parent.

Watching them become young adults is scary. It's getting harder and harder to protect them, to keep them safe from the big, complicated world of adults. I can't imagine sending them out on their own. No more than my parents could with me, I suppose.

I started university a few months after I turned sixteen. By then I had my licence, and often drove the winding roads home in the early hours of the morning, shaking off sleep. I thought I was so grown up.

My eighteenth birthday was held upstairs in my parents' hundred-year old home. The floor shook to our dancing as my parents cowered in their bedroom underneath. I remember the jeans I wore – not because I liked them but because they were always too tight around my calves. Undoubtedly I was going through a fat phase – or what I considered to be fat. I never gave myself credit, did I? Because by then I'd lost the braces and extra five kilos that I finished high school with. My pimples were clearing up. I had lots of friends and many of them had braved the dark roads of the hills to come to my party. Yep, the world was opening up.

A lot happened in the next twelve years, a whole world of living. Then it was time to have babies, and everything changed. Not in a bad way, but it took a lot of getting used to. No more putting myself first. It's a different world of living – less self-absorbed, wonderful in many ways. But with so much more to worry about.

Sometimes the angst of being a parent floors me. Not least because I see my daughters preparing to go out into the world, and I know how winding the road will be.

20 October

Every morning, my hands are so stiff that if I clench my fingers they don't touch my palms. And they're pathetically weak. Opening jars – squeezing out the dishcloth, dammit! – is a daily challenge. Any fine work with my fingers is tricky because I can't feel what I'm doing. Sometimes I burn my fingertips while cooking because it takes longer to register the heat.

If I think about it too much, I'll cry. Is this my lot – to be old before my time?

Today in my usual early morning fug, I wondered if I'd ever rock climb again. Not that I was ever a die-hard climber, but you never imagine these possibilities slipping away until one day your choices revolve around ambling walks and cups of tea.

There's something primitive about climbing. It shows you exactly what you're capable of. Or not capable of. Climbing Belougery Spire taught me the latter.

Back in my rock-climbing days, I didn't do many multi-pitch climbs, but Belougery was one of them. A pitch in climbing terms is basically as far as you can get on one rope length, around fifty metres or so. Multi-pitch climbs – of two, three or more rope lengths – must be done in stages. They're a tremendous exercise in cooperation. And trust.

But first let me explain the basics. Picture this. Two climbers at the bottom of a single-pitch cliff. One – the lead climber – has the end of the rope tied to his harness and is ready to climb. The rope connects him to the other climber, who has a belaying device on the front of her harness through which the rope runs. With a small shift of her hand, she can let the rope run smoothly through the belay device, or lock it so the rope won't move. She's secured to an anchor point by the tail end of the rope, ensuring that she can't get pulled off the ground.

As the lead climber starts ascending, she pays out the rope, making sure it stays taut between them. The lead climber pauses regularly to place protection in the rock face – generally wedges or chocks slotted into cracks – and runs his rope through these devices using a clip called a carabiner. If he slips, his partner locks the rope and his fall is arrested by the last piece of protection he put in.

When he reaches the top, he ties himself onto an anchor point, runs the rope through his own belay device, then calls to his partner that he's on belay. She disconnects the rope from her belay device, unties the bottom end of the rope from its anchor point and knots it onto her harness, then calls for her partner to pull up the slack. Once the rope is taut between them, she starts climbing, pausing to remove each piece of protection from the rock and clip it onto her harness. Her partner keeps taking in the rope as she climbs, and if she falls he locks the rope so her fall is quickly arrested. This is called top roping.

When she reaches the top, they gather up the rope and anchoring gear and walk down another route. If that's not possible, they abseil down the cliff one at a time then pull the rope down, leaving the anchoring device at the top.

Complicated, huh? With multi-pitch climbing, it gets even more so. On his ascent of the first pitch (before running out of rope), the lead climber chooses a ledge or suitable spot on the cliff to tie himself in. Then he belays his partner up to join him, and generally she continues as lead climber on the next pitch using the protective devices she collected on the climb up. In this way, they alternate leading and seconding until they reach the top of the climb.

Sorted? Now where was I? Ah, Belougery Spire.

*

My boyfriend – now my husband, so I'd better change his name – wanted to do some 'real' climbing, and I was keen too. Any excuse to go bush was good enough for me. So off we drove to the Warrumbungles and set up camp amongst a marauding mob of kangaroos. Somehow we managed to eat our meal without it being swiped by a huge buck who seemed to think we were there to feed him, then we snuggled up in our tent.

All good, a great start. But hours later in the darkness before dawn, my enthusiasm waned. I can't remember why, but at some point through the night, my bravado gave way to fear. Most of my experience was of single-pitch climbs where you can always be lowered down if you can't make the climb. This was longer than any climb I'd done – seven or eight pitches – a full day's climbing.

I decided not to do it. Max freaked. Then he cajoled. Then he freaked again. Finally he said he'd go without me and do it solo (no ropes). The fear of him dying won out, and soon we were trudging past sleeping kangaroos to Belougery.

It was a long walk. We were both sulking. As the sun started rising, we reached the bottom of the spire, an intimidating volcanic plug jutting into pastel skies. The start of the climb looked okay. Had I panicked? Max said it was fairly easy – grade fourteen, maybe fifteen tops – I'd be up in no time. I wanted to believe him, I really did.

He went up first, as usual, and I craned my head watching him move smoothly and confidently up and then across towards a ledge. Soon it was my turn. I could just see his face peering over the ledge as

I reached for the first holds. It was trickier than I expected and I misjudged a lunge and scrabbled back to the ground. Not a good start.

I dusted myself off, gave myself a stern talking to, then tried again. Success. After the first few metres, it got easier and Max smiled warmly at me as I joined him on the ledge. He busied himself tying me in and reclaiming all the bits of protection I'd retrieved ready for him to lead the next pitch. I was seconding the whole way, that was understood.

There was a slight overhang above us, enough to block my view of him as he moved on up the rock. I sat on the ledge looking out over treetops, my hands on the rope feeling for his movements and pulling in the slack.

It took me a few moments to realise what I was looking at. A koala, its lofty perch now at my eye level. I couldn't see its face clearly but it was obviously watching me. Not moving. Just staring. For several minutes, the rope jiggled but stayed tight – no doubt a tricky spot on the cliff above me – and the koala grew bored with my inactivity and turned away.

A sulphur-crested cockatoo flew towards me, its strident call echoing across the valley. I admired the gorgeous sweep of its wings in the sun and the cheeky way it braked and swung towards me, checking me out, then curved away. Bright yellow crest, crisp white wings. I smiled, loving this moment.

There was a burst of movement above, another pause and then Max's voice floated down. 'On belay, climb when ready.' My turn.

22 October

About halfway up the Spire, I lost it. I'd been trying to get up a difficult section for a while and the muscles in my hands and forearms were packing it in. I'd fallen twice, and although each time the top rope caught me, the second time Max was belaying from a point diagonally above me so I swung across the face and bashed my knee on a jutting piece of rock.

I remember the desperation rising in me. 'I want to go down!' I called, on the verge of tears.

'We can't!' yelled Max, frustrated. 'Have you looked down lately?'

I had. My stomach tightened. During our ascent, we'd been tracking diagonally across the cliff face from where we started, and not far below me the rock fell away into space. If we tried to abseil down now, we'd end up dangling in mid-air.

This is what I call a nightmare moment. Everyone has them. It's when you are absolutely trapped in an awful situation. You'd do anything to jump from that moment and find yourself in bed with tea and a book.

I was hanging from a rope halfway up a cliff and if I didn't keep climbing, we'd be stuck. Max couldn't haul me up, and he couldn't lower me down. I had no choice.

Breathe, I told myself. Keep trying. That's all I could do. I swivelled to face the view, shook my aching hands and took a few shaky breaths. The koala was down in one of those tiny trees, no doubt sitting in the same spot doing nothing. Safe and comfy. I imagined it telling me, 'Life among the treetops is pretty good. You don't have to climb a cliff just to prove yourself.' Ha, too late.

27 October

Whoa. I've been busy for days working and rushing around, and the second I stop what do I find? I'm still sad. This depression is exhausting. I could conclude that it's better to stay occupied – but isn't this how we fool ourselves? We get busy, we always have something we should be doing, distractions allowing us to skate over the surface of life.

I haven't talked about the Rosen method yet but I will – when I've finished with Belougery. But in short, it's a kind of touch therapy. I tried it once, and the therapist told me my 'should' muscles were highly developed. Ain't that the truth? If I put more energy into what I could be doing rather than what I should, I'm sure I'd be in a better place right now.

*

After my meltdown halfway up the Spire, I shook off my panic, found my holds again and finished the climb. It got easier, and by the final pitch we only had to scramble rather than climb. But by then the light was fading. Instead of worrying about getting to the top, we now had to focus on getting down.

We paused for a quick snack and drink on the narrow ridge of rock that was the peak. It was hard to enjoy the rosy late afternoon skies, knowing what was ahead. Max led the way to the other side of the Spire and we started walking down. So far, so good; no need for ropes. But in no time it was dark and as far as I can remember, we had no torches. When we came to the top of a cliff, I nearly freaked out again. Time to abseil.

Max went first and left me in the darkness, my heart pounding. A long, long pause – then his voice from below. 'Off belay.' My turn.

But I didn't seem to see in the dark as well as he could. My hands shook as I looped the rope through my belay device, running my fingers over the contours to check all was in place. Then I unclipped my protection and walked backwards over the cliff. If I'd stuffed up, I was cactus.

But I didn't die. The rope held. I abseiled down that section, then the next. Maybe even another. It was all a frightening blur. At the bottom we packed up our gear and set off on the lengthy walk back to camp. Then we dismantled our tent and drove off into the night.

The next day back at home, I checked out all my scrapes and bruises with a sense of exhilaration. I did it! But here's the catch. Here's my point.

After that climb, I couldn't go on pretending that I was brave. Or not in the way I imagined. I wasn't going to be a lead climber, and nor was I likely to do another climb like Belougery. I knew my boyfriend was disappointed in me, and that hurt.

But what hurt more was the shattering of my illusions. More thoroughly than after my fall at Ndala, when I found myself afraid of heights. I thought I'd regained my courage, I really did. I thought I was once again tough, capable Kate.

So I guess in my long-winded way I'm saying that my cancer has affected me in a similar way. It has knocked the stuffing out of me. And even though I know that I am actually pretty gutsy, that many people couldn't have climbed the Spire at all (top roping or otherwise), it's more a matter of discovering that who I thought I was is not who I am.

Who am I now?

28 October

That question plagues me. Who am I now?

It's easy to be a mother and believe that in time you'll go back to decent work and make another life for yourself once the kids have moved out.

For many years I had good reasons for not working, or working part-time, or doing jobs that fitted my parenting schedules rather than my interests. Then when my girls moved into their teens, the physical work load dropped off a bit but the emotional load intensified. Nonetheless, it got easier for me to work, and in the year before my diagnosis, I worked the most I'd done in years. But I was constantly on edge; I didn't have any spare energy. If one of my daughters asked me to help her with something after dinner, I'd be tired and crabby. On weekends I rushed around catching up on all the stuff I couldn't do through the week. I felt constantly guilty because I just wasn't there for the girls in the way I wanted to be.

Do you know that the stress hormone cortisol can affect your immune system function? In high-stress situations, cortisol stimulates the body to mobilise resources for an instant response (our 'fight or flight' reaction, protecting us from crocodiles, stampeding buffaloes… you get my drift.) But what if you're always on edge, readying yourself for a fight? Even if the attacker is a harassed boss wielding coffee-splashed budget papers, the result is the same. Constant stress leads to overproduction of cortisol, which is really bad for the immune system. And guess what? Cancer is in part due to a failure of the immune system to destroy those early cancerous cells.

Did my year of stress allow my cancer to bloom? It's not like I wasn't often stressed before that time, but the difference was that the stress was a constant presence leading up to my cancer. A buzzing in my muscles and brain – so much to do, so little time.

I'm getting sidetracked. Back to my point. I'm coming out of a long course of treatment, and also coming towards the end of years of intense parenting. I have to start thinking about me again, what I want to do for the next twenty years before I retire.

But it's not like in my twenties when I had many years ahead of me. Now my time is running out. I've got greying hair, tired skin, half a boob and a clapped out post-cancer body. And even if I wanted to throw myself back into a busy career, the spectre of that year of stress is weighing me down.

*

I'm in a bottomless pit, searching for cancer causes. Lots of maybes and could-bes and possiblys. But nonetheless here's an intriguing theory.

A while back, I heard a fascinating talk on ABC Radio National, *Rethinking our Approach to Cancer*. It was given by Paul Davies, a scientist working with the National Cancer Institute in the USA. He and his team have come up with some unusual ideas for what makes normal cells turn cancerous. This of course is the holy grail of cancer research – find out what makes the cells go AWOL in the first place and you can stop cancer in its tracks.

At this point, it occurs to me that I haven't actually explained the basics of cancer, so here's a quick summary. It starts when normal cells in a part of the body become cancerous and begin replicating themselves uncontrollably – generally forming a tumour – and eventually cells start breaking away from the tumour and entering the bloodstream. During this process of 'metastasis', the cancerous cells colonise other parts of the body and begin growing there too. These secondary tumours are what generally do most damage, especially if they're growing in vital organs.

While everyone agrees that cancerous cells are no longer normal cells, what's not clear is why they become abnormal.

The conventional theory is that random, successive mutations in cells over time lead to them becoming cancerous. Various triggers (like exposure to carcinogens, ageing and, yes, oestrogen) can hasten this mutagenic process. And while the body's immune system destroys most mutated cells, some slip through the net – especially if the immune system is compromised – or even mutate in ways that make them invisible to the immune system.

Paul Davies has some rather different ideas. He suggests that all cells have the ability to turn cancerous if the cellular environment around them is favourable. In short, his theory is that cells exposed to high-sugar, low-oxygen environments are more likely to start multiplying uncontrollably: they start acting like single-celled organisms (all out for themselves) rather than normal cells within a multicellular organism (working together for the greater good). Cancer is a complex, multi-tentacled beast, and that is one theory among many…but there's no harm in me exercising more to boost oxygen levels and reducing sugar intake, is there? Anyway, that's not what got my attention about this research. Remember me and my low iron levels? As I've said, when your body is low in haemoglobin, your blood's ability to carry oxygen is compromised, and your whole body ends up oxygen-deprived. So, for a longish time, every cell in my body was suffering low-oxygen stress. Could that be another potential cancer trigger?

I suppose it's all connected. If my high oestrogen levels caused fibroids and eventually iron deficiency, then I guess it's a moot point whether the low iron or high oestrogen (or both) might have triggered cancer. Throw in a fondness for chocolate and desserts and…argh!

Hmm, speaking of chocolate…

30 October

Remember those 'should' muscles? It sounds whacko but it makes sense. When I feel fear or dread, which muscles tighten? My stomach muscles. Anxious or worried? Forehead. Frustrated? Hands, forearms. Angry? Jaw, hands. Guilty or overly responsible? Shoulders. The muscles running from my shoulders to my neck. They're constantly ready for the things I should be doing.

I tried Rosen method therapy several months after my first seizure. I was terrified of what was going on in my head, and kept thinking my stress and anxiety must be the cause. This therapy appealed because it's about releasing the emotions and memories that get caught up in your body. Right up my alley, eh?

The Rosen method is good for people who carry long-term tension in their body. For example, imagine you have a serious accident and end up in hospital. The injuries you've sustained keep you in and out of physiotherapy rooms for years. You're doing all the right things but your back is often sore and tense. Why can't you feel healthy any more? Your body has healed but your muscles are hanging onto the memory of the accident, trying to protect you from the same thing happening again.

The therapy uses a combination of talk and touch to let your body speak up. Somehow, by touching or massaging muscles while talking, this can release the tension (trauma) being held.

So, in my endless quest to purge my demons, I went along for a trial session. It was all very civilised – lying down in a quiet, scented room and letting a softly spoken person massage my body as we chatted. I began by talking about my seizure and the woman spent some time rubbing my head. Then she started on my shoulders while I prattled on about things that were worrying me. She pointed out my 'over-developed shoulder muscles' after listening to my excuses about why my life wasn't how I wanted it to be. Poor woman.

At the end, she explained it's not unusual to feel weird after a session. She described the body as an onion, with layers and layers needing to be uncovered. It wasn't an easy or fast process.

I sat in the car for a few minutes after, trying to work out how I felt. Stirred up, yes. Better? No. My head was buzzing and my muscles jittery, not good for someone who'd recently had a grand mal seizure.

So I never went back. But sometimes I wonder what was stirred up and, if I'd gone back, where the sessions would have taken me. Like breathwork, the Rosen method exposes the bulk of the iceberg submerged beneath the tip. But I'm too impatient.

And now it seems all I've done is added more layers to the onion.

1 November

As a kid, I read fantasy and later on romance novels – escapist stuff where having special powers or a handsome lover were all that was needed to make life good. I used to hide away sometimes to read – in a comfy crook at the top of a tree, in a sunny corner of the balcony out of sight from the world. I liked imaginary worlds much more than the real world. In the real world I felt restrained. Why is that? And why am I carrying that feeling even now?

Here I am, trapped in my post-cancer body with my fears and my excuses. I've got kids, a family, a house, a life entwined with others. Every move I make is carefully considered in an effort to keep everyone happy. And me? Not so much.

If I keep feeling like this, I'll disappear in a puff of smoke.

4 November

I'm staying with a friend at the beach for a couple of nights. The sea air hums in my veins. I grew up away from the coast, but whenever I come to the water, I feel like it's home. And it's a good place to be, today.

Just over a year ago, I booked a holiday house on the coast for my daughter's birthday. It was a lovely weekend, lots of food and time to chat, read, play games. But I had a lump. I'd found it a couple of weeks before and hadn't yet done anything about it. Two weeks after that – a year ago today – I received my test results. By then, however, I'd already had my hammer blow.

After returning from the coast, I went to see my GP, who referred me for scans. I had to wait a week or so, but I wasn't too concerned. Nine out of ten breast lumps are benign – I'd be fine.

My mammogram revealed nothing, which was crazy because I could feel the lump. That's not uncommon, I was told. Then I moved on to another room for an ultrasound, where a smiling technician chatted away as she moved the ultrasound probe backwards and forwards over my lump. There it was, roundish, white and very obvious on the screen. After finishing, she called in a specialist doctor to look at the images.

He, too, was smiley and chatty. I needed a core needle biopsy of the lump – he could do it now, was that okay? I nodded, my heart gathering pace. In a flash, his instruments were out, my breast was swabbed with bright yellow antiseptic and the anaesthetic injected. After a short wait, he punched an alarmingly long needle from the right side of my breast up to the lump. He did it twice, just to be sure, wiped off the blood, said the results would take a couple of days – and gathered up his things to leave.

I pulled my gown around me and sat up hurriedly with my question. Would I need the lump removed regardless of the result? (I wanted it out, begone!)

He looked at me with his fake smile fading and then turned away to shuffle some papers. 'The next person you'll be seeing is a surgeon,' he said, his voice matter-of-fact.

'What do you mean?'

He turned to face me. 'It's cancer.'

Just like that. It's cancer.

I questioned him further as the woman who did my ultrasound busied herself in the background. He'd seen thousands of lumps, he explained. No, he couldn't be totally sure until he got the results. But he believed he was right. Then he left.

I stared at the woman as she closed my file.

'You did ask,' she said, and awkwardly patted my arm. She let me sit on the examination bed in stunned silence, but only for a minute or two. Patients to see, things to do.

Next I was out in reception, waiting for my ticket number to flash up on the screen so I could pay my several hundred dollar bill. Fuck.

I'd expected to have the tests and leave none the wiser. Instead, I left knowing my sentence. Not really believing it, not yet, but shattered nonetheless.

I sat in the car for a long time. Pain oozed out of me along with my tears. I wasn't this person, no way could this happen to me.

Dream on, girl. Three weeks later, I was in hospital with half a boob, tubes coming out of me and sickly anaesthetic on my breath.

And here I am now.

5 November

It's funny how you can get bad news – news that was always on the cards but nonetheless inconceivable when delivered – and yet continue being foolishly optimistic. I had a lump in my breast, never a good start, but I believed it would be benign. And when I found out it was cancerous, I still believed in the best-case scenario.

What the?

It was two weeks before I saw a surgeon, and by then my surgery was already booked. My surgeon – a friendly woman younger than me – was reassuring. My axillary lymph nodes (under my arm) felt normal, definitely a good sign, and the breast lump was relatively small. She said early breast cancer is highly treatable, and I was lucky I found the lump so soon. It was, however, very close to my nipple, so unfortunately I would lose that. But if I chose a lumpectomy over removal of the whole breast, my breast would be smaller but probably not much. Overall, it was a pretty good result.

Of course it all depended on what happened during surgery. She would remove and test a couple of my axillary nodes at the beginning of the surgery (sentinel node biopsy) to see if the cancer had spread. If the results were clear, she wouldn't remove any more lymph nodes. (Way better than removing them all as a precaution, which is what they used to do.) But if there was cancer in the nodes, unfortunately she'd have to take them all out. An axillary clearance, she called it.

I nodded sagely. That wouldn't happen to me.

Then on to the big question plaguing me. 'Will I need chemo?'

She smiled apologetically. Again it depended on what they found. I nodded sagely. I'd be fine.

*

Surgery day.

After a flurry of form-filling and tests, I was sent off to radiology for lymphoscintigraphy. Basically, they injected radioactive blue dye near the tumour and made me wait half an hour while it filtered through my lymph vessels to the first nodes along the line. These are the sentinel nodes, where the cancer will spread to first. Then they used a gamma-ray camera to take images of the nodes, and sent me on my way.

Several hours later, a young man appeared in the doorway of my hospital room. It was time. He wheeled my bed along the sterile corridors, joking with me as we went. Then he parked me in the surgery line-up bay, where I lay watching the operating theatre door opening and closing – people going in and out, important things happening. My anaesthetist appeared, smiling, then my surgeon with a quick but warm hello.

A bit more waiting then the anaesthetist was back. He rubbed my arm and asked if I'd like some 'bubbly'. A little treat before surgery, he said, to help relax me. 'Just like champagne!'

What could I do? I laughed and lay patiently as a nurse put a cannula in my arm and then injected the bubbly. My mood softened. Oh yes, it was nice.

Now things began to blur. The door to the operating theatre loomed large as they wheeled me in. I faintly remember the clatter of metal, bright lights, bustling activity, and…lights out.

*

When I came to, I was crying. I observed this distantly, wonderingly. Then somebody wiped the tears away and I forced myself back to wakefulness. He was nice, this nurse. I studied his strong arms and listened to his gentle voice. Then jerked fully awake.

'How many lymph nodes did they take out?'

'All of them,' he said quietly.

The tears flowed in steady waves. Oh, my god.

*

Of course there were positives. The surgery went well. The margins were clear (they removed all of the tumour). I've been told my surgeon did a great job: the scars are neat, my boob looks good (as good as can be expected). But the cancer was already spreading. My sentinel nodes were not clear. I got the axillary clearance and the chemo.

Foolish optimism, zero; dashed hopes, many.

6 November

It's not getting any better. My life. Me. Not coping, not happy, sadness just a blink away.

Today I let it all go and screamed my sorry little heart out. Oh wow, the depths. But then I heard hammering out the back and remembered that Telstra were meant to be working on the phone lines. I peeked through my tears out the back door and, sure enough, a line of orange hard hats were visible on the other side of our fence. Every window opening onto the backyard was open. They must have heard me.

OMG, the embarrassment. Except then I started to laugh. Life can turn on a dime. Or a hard hat.

12 November

I went swimming yesterday. Actual laps in a pool kind of swimming. Strangely I found the motion easier than usual, as if I've softened up somehow.

It's never been my thing, swimming. My first efforts involved thrashing around in a half empty irrigation tank while my brothers and friends threw frogs and handfuls of slime at me. Every year, we went to stay for a couple of weeks by the beach but it was always midwinter – the only time my parents could leave the orchard for an extended period. We'd go where the southern ocean spumed high against granite headlands, and I'd spend hours with my siblings trawling rock pools, digging in the sand, fishing, fighting. We never swam.

It would be years before I ventured into big seas. In my late teens, I went to the fabled Manly Beach in Sydney that I'd heard so much about. The waves were crammed with people so I figured I'd be all right. I managed to dislodge my bikini top a couple of times when dumpers caught me but the surf can't have been that big because I was embarrassed but never scared.

Several years later, again in Sydney, I swam out after my boyfriend (yep, the same one) in wild seas at Dee Why beach. I knew you had to duck dive under the bigger waves to avoid being dumped, and soon I was out the back of the breakers with all the surfers. Max was impressed to see me there, and I soon found out why.

A set came through and the surfers cleared out: paddling further out to sea or catching one of the smaller waves in to shore. I was left in no-man's-land with Max trying to tell me what to do. He couldn't help me much.

I didn't know how to bodysurf, and I wasn't a strong swimmer or diver. I ducked under one wave, and came up gasping for breath just in time to face the next. My feeble effort at diving under this one took me straight into the washing machine cycle from hell.

When it spat me back to the surface, an even bigger wave loomed above me. This one creamed me, good and proper. I was powerless – tossed around like seaweed with my empty lungs shrieking at me to do something.

Luckily, it was the last wave in the set. My feet met sand and I staggered through the whitewash and lay down on the shore. I was spray-painted with sand, my hair was clogged with it, and it dribbled from my nose in a trail of snot.

After that, I wouldn't go out in big surf. Max tried many times, and railed at my fear. He wanted me to be a gutsy surfer chick, I guess.

In my usual manner, I chose to ignore this new piece of knowledge about myself. I imagined that farm girl (tough girl) Kate would reassert herself and I'd be out in the surf in no time. But I never went out in big waves again. And after a mere thirty years, I've finally worked out why. It's partly about being suffocated and overwhelmed. And more than anything it's about loss of control. My greatest fear.

No wonder cancer has hit me so bad.

13 November

During my swim at the pool the other day, my right arm started to go tingly for the last lap or so. I knew my underarm still wasn't normal from the surgery but to have the whole arm play up surprised me. Furthermore, after ten laps my back muscles felt weary in a way they never used to.

My body is so weak now.

Last night, I dreamt I saw myself in the mirror, and my legs were a horror show: a long, crumpled scar ran down my right thigh and the flesh above and below was shrunken and disfigured as if burnt. My upper thighs were bulging with flabby lumps, a sort of caricature of fatness you'd never see in real life.

It's funny the ways dreams distort things, picking out the essence of a feeling or experience and expanding on it. That scar on my leg looked like a bigger and much uglier version of the one on my breast. People say my scar is neat and nicely healed, but to disfigure a breast is to lose what society defines as beautiful.

Swimming reminded me of my weakness. Of my scars.

I used to pride myself on my strength. My physique is naturally quite powerful: I have broad shoulders, a strong back and muscly legs. A childhood spent playing sport, riding my horse and working on the orchard in holidays accentuated this.

For some reason, I needed to be strong. I used to measure myself against my brothers with arm wrestles and show-off tree climbing. At uni, I glowed when my friends commented on my well-developed biceps. On bushwalks, I prided myself on staying up front, proving how accomplished I was.

What was that all about? I guess it doesn't matter. What matters now is that another of my supports is crumbling, and I don't know how to hold myself up. Not yet.

17 November

My dishwasher has taught me a lesson. It's not a very good dishwasher. Even on a long cycle, you have to rinse dishes before you put them in. But for a while now I've been using the shortest cycle to save power. With the superduper dishwasher tablets, it works okay, but everything has a slight soapy residue. With the cheaper tablets, it works badly and still leaves a soapy residue. And yet I keep trying different brands of tablets and convincing myself I can keep using the short cycle.

Yesterday I had to rewash at least a third of the dishwasher's contents after a wash, which kind of defeats the purpose, doesn't it? But as I scrubbed coffee granules off a plate, it dawned on me that this was my pattern. Despite overwhelming evidence to the contrary, I fool myself that 'next time will be different'. It's the classic sticking my head in the sand routine.

And it's what I'm doing now. Things don't always turn out for the best… I know that. But what have I changed? Not a lot.

Sure, I'm eating healthily, I rarely drink alcohol and I'm not rushing around like a headless chook in the way I was. My treatments should have blitzed my cancer, and if high oestrogen levels were involved in my getting sick, they're no longer an issue (menopause and hormonal therapy having put paid to all that).

What's not changing is my attitude: my regular focus over the years on what's wrong with my life. Did that added stress sap the cancer fighting energy out of me? Is it now?

I don't know the answer, and if I go back to my biological

ramblings about the world being a threatening place regardless of how well we try to protect ourselves, again I'll conclude that a stress-free life is not our due.

There's no free ride, even now when life is much safer (for most people anyway). When I look around me, I see people on edge, trying to make do in a crazy modern world. Feeling overwrought for months on end is more usual than not, wouldn't you say? So I can hardly lay claim to being more stressed or emotionally troubled than most of my brethren. And in my limited experience, do I see cancer singling out those who are more unhappy, or have more troubles in life? It doesn't appear to.

So there, I'm talking myself out of the stress=cancer theory.

But when I think about my year of stress leading up to my cancer diagnosis, there's no doubt this was a new level of anxiety for me. Was this the point at which it all got too hard for my body? Even if stress wasn't the cause, was it the final straw? I'm hardly in a position to dismiss that possibility.

Having cancer is forcing me out of my complacency. I'm not young any more. My options are narrowing, year by year. If I want to be happier with myself and my life, I really can't put off doing something about it any longer.

When I think about what I need to change, I keep coming back to this: I like who I am. My problem is not so much changing who I am, but swapping my focus from what's wrong, to what's right.

On the weekend, an old friend came to stay. She was telling me of a walk she'd done recently up to a lighthouse in Sydney, which reminded her of when I'd taken her and her boyfriend rock climbing there years before.

I'd forgotten that. For all my talk of not being brave enough to do lead climbing, and not being keen on multi-pitch climbs – here was my friend reminding me I was proficient enough to set up a top rope and instruct two beginners on how to climb a cliff safely.

So here's an alternative interpretation. I was a good climber.

Flexible, strong, determined. When the going got tough, I struggled, but always pulled through. I didn't like taking risks, and that's okay.

How's that?

18 November

The past keeps tapping at my shoulder. Gently reminding me of who I once was. Today, my mind is on my university days.

When I started uni, I couldn't believe how right it felt. This was where I was meant to be. On orientation day, the uni lawns were crowded with students encouraging people to join their clubs. There were no teachers keeping tabs on people. Nobody wore uniforms. Everyone wanted to be there. And there were boys everywhere. I'd spent five uneasy years in an all-girls school, and being back in a unisex world felt natural.

After checking out what activities were on offer, I signed up to play squash and joined the science and mountaineering clubs. I was away!

While the Science Club turned out to be mostly about drinking, squash was a great choice. I've played it off and on for years. But it was the Mountain Club that really captured my soul. I'd been camping once with my family in the Flinders Ranges and loved it, so bushwalking – hiking for days with a backpack – promised to be just my thing.

Upcoming walks were posted on the club noticeboard. All you had to do was put your name on the list before it filled up and you were in. I signed up for a trip to Mount Falkland in the Flinders Ranges, and offered myself up as a driver. Then I borrowed a backpack and sleeping bag, bought a sleeping mat and some boots, and was hot to trot.

The weeks at uni whizzed by and on the first day of the Easter break my new Mountain Club friends and I hit the highway. My trusty little car wallowed under the weight of five people and their backpacks. Semi-trailers blasted dust and diesel fumes through the open windows but we didn't care.

This was the sort of adventure I'd been waiting for.

19 November

A year ago today, I was in hospital waiting for surgery. One year since the intervention truly began.

When I saw my oncologist a couple of weeks after my surgery, he jollied me along by saying, 'This time next year, you'll be over it all. You'll really enjoy your Christmas.'

Well, I'm over it all. Completely over it.

It feels like every time I try to go back to normal I trip up. This time it's my neck. Was it sweeping up leaves? Climbing onto the roof to clean the gutters? Whatever did it, I spent half of last night awake, trying to find a position in bed where my neck didn't hurt. And now I'm sitting in front of my computer monitor because it's the only position where I can sit with my back supported and do stuff without looking down.

When is it going to end?

And as for Christmas, the thought of presents, celebrations and expectations makes me want to cry. Last Christmas, I was a shadow person: a week past my first chemo dose, plodding along waiting for my hair to fall out and wishing the next year away. This year, what am I?

When in doubt, go back to the past again.

*

Mount Falkland. My first bushwalking trip.

By early afternoon, we'd positioned cars at either end of our route, distributed food and water between everyone's packs and were walking off into the dry inland.

The Flinders Ranges is an amazing place. It's all red rocks and blue skies. Creeks are often just a series of stagnant rock pools and waterfalls rarely live up to their names. Our route was carefully planned around water sources and, because these were dubious at best, we carried water purification tablets so we'd have something safe to drink.

As the warm autumn air started to cool, we set up camp. There's something magical about how a group of people can turn a grassy clearing into a cosy campground. We didn't bother with tents – just spread camp mats on the ground and fluffed our sleeping bags onto them. In no time, wood was gathered and a fire lit in a ring of stones. Pots filled with discoloured creek water were ready for our feast – tuna mornay followed by packet cheesecake and smoky billy tea.

This was where the trip really began. We sat up for hours with the inland air cold on our backs, telling stories, laughing, getting to know each other better. The Milky Way spanned the glittering sky above us. Animals rustled in nearby bushes and every so often rocks clattered as someone vanished into the darkness to relieve themselves.

I loved the simplicity of it all. Normal life receded and the basics took over. Water, food, warmth, company.

20 November

People often ask am I 'clear' of cancer, have I had all the scans and blood tests to show all's fine? Well, it's not that easy. There's no blood test, not much they can look for. I go for regular check-ups with specialists and have annual breast scans. That's it. All I can do is wait. And hope.

I suppose I could insist on full body and bone scans like I had a year ago, but they're expensive. It's an equation – does the low likelihood of recurrence justify the high expense and invasiveness of ongoing scans?

No need to overreact. I'm sure I'll be okay. Except I can't trot that one out any more.

This morning, I went for my annual breast scans. Something to look forward to each year. I was booked in for a mammogram first. In a tiny cubicle, I stripped from the waist up, donned my hospital gown and sat on the bench, fidgeting. A young woman ushered me into a drab room with the blinds down. In the middle of the room was a machine, rather old-looking, with large flat X-ray plates attached to a rotating arm. Off came the gown (why do they bother?), at which point the woman saw my chest and realised she'd made a faux pas by asking if it was my first time. She got me to stand pushed up against the machine with my left boob loaded onto a flat plate and an arm draped awkwardly along the edge of the machine. Next she lowered the top plate and squeezed my breast into a focaccia shape, then ducked behind a protective screen and pushed the nuke button. Back she came for a new position – a vertical focaccia this time. After that, it was time to squish my sorry excuse for a right boob between the plates. I nearly fainted.

My torturer left me sitting on a chair staring glumly at the X-ray machine and went to find a doctor to check the scans. She bustled back in, smiling. One more, that's all! Back in the machine went my left boob, this time with the plates tilted on an angle. Another pause while she got the new scan checked.

Finally I got the all-clear. Time to return to my cubical to sit and ponder life. I reminded myself that my lump didn't even show up on last year's mammogram. It was the ultrasound that would reveal my fate.

'Catherine?' came my summons through the door. My full name, rarely used until recently.

The baby-faced ultrasound dude ushered me into another darkened room, and asked me to lie down with my gown slipped off my right shoulder. Funny, these attempts to allow people their modesty. I'm too old to worry about strange young men seeing my breasts – especially ones like mine. And no doubt this guy has seen it all before.

Squelch went the warm gel all over my skin, then he started running a hand-held ultrasound probe over my skin. He pushed quite hard and it hurt my mammogram-squashed flesh. I watched on the screen overhead as he passed the probe backwards and forwards over the same spot near my armpit. My heart picked up pace. On the screen, two small lumps like coffee beans.

He moved away, making methodical sweeps over the rest of my breast. Then he returned to the coffee beans. The keyboard and mouse clicked as he drew boxes and arrows, and took endless images from different angles.

I lay quietly panicking. Seeing it all. Mastectomies, more chemo, months of trauma to come. Holy crap.

He handed me a towel to wipe off the gunk, then asked me to cloak the right side and bare the left. More methodical sweeps were done and finished in no time.

'Um, I'd like to have another look at the right side. Just to be sure.'

NO!

As the gel glooped down again, I gathered courage. 'What are those two lumps you were looking at?'

'I'm sure one is a lymph node. The other is probably one too.'

Lymph nodes? He must've heard the breath puff out of me.

'Oh, is it normal to have them in the breast?' (Why hadn't I seen them on my first ultrasound?)

'Sure.'

Hmm.

Off he went to get a doctor. Who repeated the scanning (again pushing too hard) while talking gobbledygook to the ultrasound technologist.

Then the doctor smiled down at me. 'We're almost certain they're normal lymph nodes. But just to be sure, come back in five or six months for another scan. However, if you're worried I can biopsy them for you?'

No. Way.

I scurried off home to recover.

26 November

After giving my dog Chico his treat this morning, I stood in the sun enjoying my surrounds. The air had that stillness which heralds a hot day, and the birds were busy in our fruit trees making the most of the early cool. I breathed in the good energy around me and felt it flowing through my body like water on a dried up salt lake.

*

That bushwalk to Mount Falkland had it all: romance, adventure, drama...

For starters, it was when I met my first boyfriend. He was obviously keen on me, and so was another guy. Yep, I found myself playing the field. My new friend Karen was keen on guy #2, who seemed interested in her too. So there was a little bit of rivalry going on there.

Despite her relaxed personality, Karen had a medical condition which meant she bruised easily and bled profusely from even small cuts. Although it didn't seem to worry her much, we were all protective of her. After two days of walking, her legs were a mess of bruises in various shades and red scratches, and someone hit on the name Nougat. She liked it.

Reaching the top of Mt Falkland was a rush. I dropped my heavy, sweaty pack and felt the lifting of my shoulders, the slowing of my breath. We stood there looking out over paradise, handing around chocolate mint slices and laughing and chatting. How good is that?

I can't remember if we camped up there, but what I do remember is walking down from the peak with dark rainclouds closing in on us. The deluge came quickly – sluicing the dry earth into mud and turning gullies into streams. We slithered down, unbalanced by our packs, anxious to escape. Sean (guy #2) kept close by Karen, helping her down slippery sections.

At the bottom, there was no time for rest. The rain fell relentlessly, and the desert around us swelled with water.

After a while, we came to a creek, undoubtedly dry just a few hours before but now running fast. The rain had backed off a little so we paused for a drink and scroggin (fruit, nuts and lollies, yum). We watched the water streaming off the hillsides into the creek, and mused about the possibility of a flash flood. Time to get going.

My (soon-to-be) boyfriend, Rudi, and a couple of others started looking for the best way to cross the creek, and yelled for us to follow them a little way upstream. As they picked their way across some large boulders, we heard a sound. A distant rumble swelling rapidly to a roar.

'Flash flood!' someone screamed.

'Get across the creek!' I added, pointlessly.

Rudi and the other two bounded across to the far bank as the flood came at them. A metre-high wall of brown, debris-filled water engulfed the rocks they'd just crossed over and roared past us with frightening power. We all watched, gobsmacked. This was the stuff of movies.

The water subsided a little, but the new level was much higher. Sticks and logs sailed past, swirling and bashing into rocks. But we had no choice, we had to cross.

We held our breaths as Karen had her turn. Sean – a solid, powerful guy – was right by her, taking her pack and making sure she didn't slip. But she was okay. We were all okay.

Soon we were on our way again – boots squelching, water dripping in our wake. We reached an old fire trail and our spirits rose as the clouds lifted. Rudi walked beside me, and as we talked I felt his hand reach tentatively for mine. Ah.

At some point, I looked behind and there were Karen and Sean holding hands too.

*

That wasn't the end of our adventure, but I'll speed up the story. We made it back to Sue's car, parked near an old homestead marking the end of our walk. The group set up for the night on the homestead veranda while I left with Sue to retrieve my car from where I'd parked it at the beginning of our walk. But the route to my car was along the bottom of a winding gorge and Sue struggled to get her car through the flooded creek crossings, bashing the underside on rocks and nearly getting bogged. I took over for a while but at a particularly nasty-looking crossing we stopped, defeated. What now?

Our rescuer came in the form of a National Park ranger in a hefty four-wheel drive. You beauty! He towed us through the crossing then escorted us onwards, his tow rope at the ready. We couldn't believe our luck.

When we reached my car, I jumped out and kissed it. But now the light was fading, and the ranger advised us to drive to a nearby town and wait out the flood till morning.

The next day, refreshed after a pub meal and a soft bed, we made a lengthy detour around the flooded areas and found an easier way in to retrieve our friends. They were damp and smelly after a night spent on a cold veranda while we were clean and smug. Oh yes.

*

One of the great things about growing up is learning what you're capable of. That first bushwalk showed me I coped well with difficult situations. I could lug my pack through rugged terrain and sleep on hard ground; I could wade across treacherous streams and drive through flooded creek crossings.

When I went through my cancer treatment, people complimented me on being so strong. I'd laugh off such statements – I certainly didn't feel strong at the time – but looking back I see that I was.

Hold on to that.

10 December

Let me talk about Tamoxifen. As I've explained, it's an essential part of the breast cancer treatment regime for someone like me. A tiny substance bumping around my circulatory system, making its way to my breast cells and camping in their oestrogen receptors. Getting in the way so oestrogen can't kick start the cancer cycle again.

All women know, however, that oestrogen affects mood. Blocking the effects of oestrogen is bound to have consequences.

Soon after finishing radiotherapy, I started taking my pills, confident that it was what I needed. As the weeks passed, my mood plummeted. I tried convincing myself that this sludge settling in my soul would eventually dissipate. That I'd be able to move on.

Not so.

People kept reminding me I'd been through a lot. It's normal to struggle with depression and feeling overwhelmed. 'So much to deal with! Such a shock to the body! Give it time. You'll be okay.' Yah de yah.

I know me. I know my own peculiar versions of sadness and depression. Yes, it's true there has been a lot going on – I've had plenty of reasons to feel down. I don't pretend that without Tamoxifen I'd have been deliriously happy. But this blanketing greyness? This inability to cope on so many levels? Not me.

In early November, I could barely stand it. I cut back to one Tamoxifen pill every two days. And sure enough, by the end of November, the bleakness had started to lift. Just a bit, enough to show me I wasn't imagining things.

My conviction grew that I couldn't be this Tamoxifen person. It was disabling. So a week ago I bustled along to see my oncologist, prepared for a bit of a confrontation. I needed an alternative, even if it was just to maintain a reduced dose.

Fifteen minutes later, I bounced out the door, grinned at the receptionist and skipped down to the car. My oncologist had agreed that I couldn't go on like this. He told me to stop taking Tamoxifen, and to return in January for a blood test to check my hormonal levels. If this shows I've been through menopause, that's it. No more Tamoxifen!

What a funny way to celebrate menopause.

16 December

I'm staying with my elderly parents until the end of the month. There's a lot going on in their lives, and much of it is difficult and upsetting. But right now they're absorbed in something outside of themselves. They're sitting upstairs watching the aftermath of a siege in Sydney. A café full of shoppers and office workers was in lockdown for a day, a gunman holed up inside with his coffee-drinking hostages. Big chunks of the city centre were evacuated. The media gobbled up the drama and regurgitated it as day-long news feeds and interviews. My parents sat around watching television for hours yesterday, and now they're watching it again. Three people died, including the gunman. He's been pronounced a lone wolf, a nutter – nothing to worry about. Don't be fearful people.

But it's true, we shouldn't be. For all the terrible things that happen around us, most people in Australia get old. My parents are eighty-five and eighty-six. And at their age, not much happens. They struggle with the simple tasks of living: a doctor's appointment is an event now rather than an annoyance. So these unfolding dramas on TV? A reminder of the bigger world out there. Of the greater community they were once so entangled with.

And today, of all days, they might need distracting from their memories. Yes, I said most of us will get old. But Michael didn't. And today is his birthday.

I'm not sure if my parents know the date, and it's not something I'd mention. The loss of a child – there's no plastering over that wound. It's not something you 'get over'. The scar remains, jagged and ugly. But these days, my parents seem less affected by the awfulness that life can dish out. I'd been dreading telling them I had breast cancer, but when I finally did they weren't particularly shocked or upset, just kind of surprised. Their response was underwhelming. Death, sickness, tragedy – all too familiar to them. Too much to get hung up on any more. Much better to let it all grow dim in memory.

So perhaps forgetfulness is one of nature's small mercies. As we grow older and feebler, the memories piling in our wake lose their hold. They become mystical rather than raw.

*

Michael's birthday. If he was still alive, he'd be forty-seven, greying or balding, a little rounder around the middle perhaps. We'd have forgotten the person he was at twenty-one. But now he's frozen in time as a gangly youth, barely a man, with a wry smile trapped on his lips. I see him as he is in photos – how cruel is that? Why can't my mind conjure him up as a video replay? Or maybe that will come as I get older – a brief chance to relive my youth before I too join the shadows.

But even if the images are blurry, here's something I remember. He was a dreamer and gathered knowledge to fuel his dreams. *National Geographic* magazines littered his room. He'd lie on his bed for hours, reading and smoking. Then he'd appear in the kitchen chewing minty gum, which always made me laugh. No doubt everyone knew he smoked.

I'm sure, given time, he'd have found his way to Route 66 and driven that highway in some big old Pontiac or Chevrolet, a cigar in his hand and sunshine in is his face.

*

A couple of days ago, my twin brother told me a story. When he was younger, he slept in one of the two dingy rooms above the old stables up the driveway. By then, there were spare rooms in my parents' house, but Marty liked where he was.

The room adjacent to his was empty, but years before it had been Mike's. On the last morning of his life, Mike stepped down from that room and drove to his lonely outpost above the city where he took his life.

So early one morning years later, Marty was sleeping in his room above the stables when his new girlfriend woke him up. She'd seen someone, she said, sitting on the end of their bed. A young guy, tall, with short-cropped hair. He was wearing jeans and work boots. Marty asked what top he had on and she described what I call a grandpa shirt – checked pattern, soft flannelette fabric. In short, she described Mike. As soon as Marty gave me this description, I could see him there, sitting on the bed. It had to be him.

Sceptics would say she'd seen a photo of Mike and dreamt she saw him. Maybe. But Marty says she hadn't seen any photos.

I believe it was him, of course I do. But why did he appear to her while Marty, his brother, slept on? And why didn't Mike come sit on my bed?

But as I type I can see him in my mind, shaking his head with that wry grin. The answer is simple: he knows how it would smart in our souls. To see him like that would bring the memories flaring back into the present, and forever after we'd be watching for him, waiting for his reappearance. Imagine if he did that to my parents. Their angst would be reignited. Magnified. It wouldn't be fair.

But oh – to see him just once!

Happy birthday, Mike. I miss you still.

20 December

This time last year, I was on day 2 post-chemo. Popping my anti-nausea pills, monitoring my body to see how it would manage the toxic load in my veins. I felt vague and antsy at the same time – my thoughts flattened by chemicals, my body buzzing with steroids and the as yet unrecognised side effects of the anti-nausea drug Maxolon. My body fluctuated from slightly overheated to hot, my head was pretty much hot all the time. Hot flushes came when I lay down, sat up, stood up, sat down – and frequently in between. My limbs were puffy with fluid. Coffee, herbal teas, alcohol, sugary foods – all tasted unpleasant. My mouth was tender, so I couldn't have hot food or drinks. I craved raw vegies and simple foods – had to have them – but was nonetheless constipated. I was tired but slept erratically and badly.

But all up, believe it or not, it was manageable. I was pleased about that.

Back then it was all about coping with the shorter-term side effects. Some came and went with each cycle, some lingered for weeks or months after I finished chemo. What I hadn't anticipated are the ones that are still with me.

I've a friend going through chemo. She had her second dose a week ago. It's been tough – after her first round, she ended up in hospital with a critically low white blood cell count and multiple infections. This time, she's been dosed with a drug to give her white blood cell production a boost, and she's avoided hospital. But she has mouth and sinus infections, a bitter metallic taste in her mouth, and no doubt a host of other side effects she's not mentioning.

Unlike me, she didn't find a lump. So her first intimation that something was wrong was during a routine mammogram. Suddenly she was being whisked off for an ultrasound and biopsy, and not long after she was on her way home with a probable diagnosis ringing in her ears. Cancer.

So yay, chemo will do the trick for her too. It's worth the horribleness.

Although she won't see this as a positive, at least she's in the bosom of the medical profession. Her life is being managed by others and she can relax into that – for the moment. But once she steps off the conveyor belt in a few months' time, there'll be no going back to normal.

At my end of the ride, there's no happy ending. No certainty that it won't happen again. And there's the cloying knowledge that physically I am damaged. Not in ways that other people can see (unless I bare my broken breast). It's in my wilted vitality, my creaky joints, my bruised soul.

So many flow-on effects I hadn't thought of. Like with my dad. His memory is failing, and several times during my stay he's told me that he knows who I am but can't believe I'm his daughter. If you asked him what he did an hour ago, he might remember if it was something he was stimulated by, but the next day he'd most likely have forgotten. Most of his living is vanishing into a mist, so he has to rely on old memories. And his memory of me is of someone with shoulder-length red hair. So when I turn up with short blonde hair, he can't place me. This new Kate doesn't fit in his memory bank and can't be added to it.

Just another thing.

13 January

I'm back at home and it's a new year. Happy New Year! And surely it must be.

But how hard it is to be 'positive'. That's the advice people keep giving me. Easy to say the words, guys, but how do I make it happen? What guarantees do I have?

None.

Today I'm thinking not of where I've been but of where I could be now. When I had surgery, stray cancer cells were already making their way from my breast out into the unchartered waters of my healthy body. If I'd discovered that lump only today, my story might have ended quite differently.

So what is my story? The phoenix rising from the ashes? Kate going out into the world armed with her shiny shield. 'I survived cancer, I can survive anything.'

Nope. Not me. It takes so little to knock me. Two days ago, I mowed the lawn and stopped halfway for a cry. It was so hard. Yesterday, I had an easy hit of squash and now I hurt all over. I'm worn to the core.

And yet, I feel my spirit returning. As the chemicals, all of them, drain from my system, I feel the essence of me returning. Slowly, shakily – but she's there. The person I value and love. She's been buried for a while but thankfully, she's still there. Hello!

22 January

Who was I kidding?

I went back to my oncologist yesterday to get the lowdown on my menopausal status and continuing treatment. Where does it leave me?

Crushed.

Let's start with my blood test last week. Because of my surgery, I can't have blood taken from my right arm. There's a risk of infection and therefore lymphoedema (damage to the lymph vessels). That leaves my left arm – the one with all the chemo-trashed veins.

When I went for the test, I sat in the big chair and tried not to think of the last time someone stuck a needle in me: during my final round of chemo, when my veins were such a mess it took four goes to get the cannula needle in. But that was nine months ago. Surely my veins were much better now?

I looked away as the nurse picked up the finest needle she could find and gently pushed it into my forearm. Then she pushed harder.

And harder. At last the needle popped through the scarred walls of my vein. I gritted my teeth, waiting for the blood to start flowing. The nurse sighed, jiggled the needle slightly, sighed again and started moving the needle around more firmly. I winced, she apologised.

'Ah,' she said. 'Got it.'

We watched the dark fluid move into the syringe, then stop.

A long pause, then another sigh. 'I'm really sorry but it's not flowing.' She pulled out the needle and pushed a wad of gauze onto my damaged arm.

I winced again.

She rubbed the back of my hand. 'I might have to put the needle in a vein there,' she said and I felt a trickling of nausea through my system. This was way too close to my chemo experience.

Thankfully she chose another vein in my forearm and I steeled myself as the needle crunched through the vein wall and into my bloodstream. I leaned back, fighting a wave of sickness.

Another pause, another jiggle, another pause.

Then, 'Don't move a muscle!'

As dark blood began filling the syringe, spots appeared in my vision. My heart raced, my skin was clammy. Breathe, breathe, I told myself through the nausea and panic.

At last it was done. I walked out, still shaky. Surprising how quickly I could find myself back there in the chemo ward. Sickening.

But a week later – back to my more optimistic self – I walked calmly into my oncologist's room. Deliverance day? No.

He studied my blood test results with a frown and my heart sank. 'Well,' he said, looking up, 'you're definitely through menopause. But that's the least of our concerns.'

What? Last time he said menopause was a key part of the treatment. Why was it suddenly less vital?

He clicked to another window on his computer and started reading again.

I monitored myself, wondering why I was so miserable. I'd been expecting this result; hoping for it even. But now the menopause genie was out of the bottle, I felt alarmingly upset. Cancer had taken my vitality from me, my sexuality, and now my status as a fertile woman. At forty-eight years, this should hardly be a concern – surely I'd been on the cusp of menopause anyway. But somehow I'd traversed menopause and barely noticed it. The loss of periods, the hot flushes, the moodiness and depression – all quite probably attributable to chemo, radiation, hormonal treatment. Menopause itself was a non-event. And now here I was, a woman with dead ovaries on the wrong side of life. It totally sucked.

And of course there was more. I'd been fooling myself thinking I might be finished with hormonal therapy.

My oncologist explained that as Tamoxifen was no longer right for me, it was time to start taking aromatase inhibitors. This class of hormonal therapy drugs has lower side effects than Tamoxifen, but is only effective after menopause. Now I was through the change, lucky me, I could move on to these 'better' drugs, which he recommended I take for five years.

I stared at a photo on the wall as he cranked out the statistics. Even in my post-menopausal state, the chance of my cancer recurring was still 1 in 3. If I took the drugs? 1 in 6.

Way too convincing.

I'd already done some reading about aromatase inhibitors (AIs). While Tamoxifen works by occupying oestrogen receptors on cells, AIs go a step further. They stop the production of oestrogen by interfering with the action of the aromatase enzyme which produces oestrogen. But the end result is the same – a kind of chemical castration, for a very good cause.

Of course there's no free ride with drugs. My oncologist cited bone thinning (osteoporosis), heart problems and joint pain as possible side effects – along with depression, of course. He urged me to give AIs a go, and if I felt really bad, I could stop taking them. At least then I'd have tried everything.

Fair enough?

*

I went home, did some googling and added more side effects from aromatase inhibitors. Memory problems, anxiety, trouble sleeping, hot flushes, night sweats, hair thinning, numbness and tingling in hands/fingers, swelling of limbs, tiredness, dizziness, headaches, nausea, liver dysfunction, constipation/diarrhoea, weight gain…

These were all just possibilities, I knew that. Read the fine print for any medication and there's always a worrying list of potential side effects.

But these ones rang alarm bells.

- Heart problems? When I was iron-deficient, I had heart palpitations, and they had returned while I was on Tamoxifen.
- Numbness/tingling in fingers? I already had that.
- Joint pain? My hip joints had started playing up since taking Tamoxifen.
- Memory problems? No way! I had too many of those already.
- Osteoporosis, hair thinning? Talk about putting me on an express train to old age.

All that aside, the last thing I needed was to be weighed down for years to come by a heavy cloak of pessimism, bleakness, depression. Every cell in my body screamed NO.

I pushed aside my laptop and cried. The pain of it cascaded through me, taking me right back to the beginning of it all. I'd been lifted, slightly, by holidays and the cessation of Tamoxifen treatment. But now here I was, back in that dreadful (dreading) place where I was trapped with nowhere to go. Weighing bad outcomes against badder ones.

What was I doing with *cancer*?

24 January

I rang Dad today for his birthday. He's eighty-six – a distinguished age indeed.

He was chirpy and said lots of people had been ringing and saying nice things. But then he confessed he wasn't sure who they were, even though he knew they must be family members. And he kept asking me how old he was.

When we're younger, we think that making it to eighty-six is a great achievement. And so it is, really. But tell that to my dad as he struggles with his failing memory and confusion. In his heart, he's still a young guy with the world ahead of him.

But enough of that.

My dad is what I'd call a typical older-generation Aussie bloke. A fix-it man with strong hands and calloused fingers. He shows his love by doing stuff, by helping in practical ways. When I was a teen, he used to grizzle about me having a horse, but on the weekends he'd grab his tools and follow me up the hill for the latest repair job: a faulty water tank float or yet another hole in the galvanised iron of the horse shed. (My sister's horse used to corner my horse inside the shed and bite him, and a couple of times Prince kicked his hoof right through the iron.)

I remember one day I was helping Dad put up the wire fence around the horse paddock, and Dad was tightening the wire by winding it round and round a short but thick tree branch. Something happened – perhaps he slipped – and he lost his grip. The branch spun from his hand and cracked him on the side of the head. I still remember the thud it made against his skull

He shouted in pain and bent over with his head in his hands, all the time releasing a string of expletives. I knew this meant he'd be okay, because whenever he hurt himself he swore like a trooper. Even from across the gully, we all knew about it when he hit his finger while hammering, or grazed his shin with an errant piece of kindling while chopping wood.

When finally he straightened up, his face was bright red and his eyes were brimming, but he didn't cry. He told me he was all right and returned to the fence.

When I look at Dad now, even though his spine has collapsed from years of hard work (reducing him from six feet tall to my height), he still has those hands. Big and strong, marked by life. I love those hands.

What I also love is how Dad has become more emotional with age – in a good way. When I was young, he was simply too busy to allow his emotions much play. We all knew he was a big softie, underneath the sometimes gruff exterior, but in the last twenty years he's become gentler. Not that long ago, he'd ring me sometimes and tell me of books or movies which had moved him to tears. And he'd send me photos of the orchard, with autumn leaves bright against green hillsides, or of the house in spring surrounded by fruit trees dense with blossoms. I've a little album in my bedside table which he sent me several years back, full of photos from home because he knows I miss it.

Happy birthday, Dad. I love you.

1 February

Today's Decision Day. I've had more than a week to stew, and it's this simple. No matter the medical recommendations, no matter my fear of recurrence, it seems I can't do it. I can't take an aromatase inhibitor, can't subject myself to more chemicals. My passive treatment days are over, now it's time to take control.

2 February

Taking control, huh? Not easy given the overwhelming loss of control I've experienced over the last year or so – but I think it's about trusting myself. My response until now has been to keep hoping somebody will hand me the solution. But it's not coming. No treatment provides guarantees. No medico or alternative therapist has all the answers.

My decision to refuse ongoing treatment with aromatase inhibitors is scary, but weirdly empowering. It really is up to me now.

*

Despite all my theories, I'll never know why I got cancer. But there are things I can do to protect myself. Time to supercharge my diet, exercise more, de-stress when I can, avoid nasty chemicals… In short, I need a staying healthy security blanket to tide me over this scary patch.

I've come up with a plan, which started as a list but turned into a dissertation, so I've stuck it on at the end.

5 February

More birthdays. This time it's my oldest daughter's. Eighteen, who'd have thought? (My life measured by the age of my kids – 'tis the ageing parents' refrain.)

This is her gap year and she's saving up for an extended trip overseas. My first baby – now not a baby at all – is confident, full of life and ready to get on with it. She'll be fine. But thinking about her going away makes me queasy, I can't help it.

At her age, it's natural to scoff at fretting parents – I did the same – but now the shoe is on the other foot. Nearly twenty years of caring is a long, long time. There's no doubt I will fuss and flap around her before she leaves, and lie awake night after night once she's gone. But how fabulous that she's doing this.

Happy birthday, my baby girl grown big. You are a miracle. I love you from the bottom of the sea to the stratosphere and beyond.

9 February

How rarely do I see the night. Smell it. Feel it.

Last night, I went walking with my oldest daughter and a friend. There's a large bush reserve near my house and a fire trail smooth enough to walk along in the dark without tripping.

It was a warm evening, partly cloudy, and the moon hadn't risen, so the stars were bright. As we walked I looked up at the Southern Cross and the nearby Pointers, and used bisecting lines from both to locate south (a little trick I learnt from my boyfriend at uni). I wondered how many times I'd done this over the years – during nights spent lying in my sleeping bag out bush with no tent over me, or sitting with my back to a hot campfire and watching the sky. Soaking in the cool, impassive gaze of the stars and remembering my place in a wider world.

Last night felt like therapy. Breathing in, absorbing the night and the silent stars. Feeling the goodness. It confirmed what I should know but keep forgetting: nature is part of my cure.

As if to prove a point, when I went outside later to see my friend off, I noticed the sky was lighter above the bush reserve. 'The moon must be rising,' I said.

We crossed the road to get a better view and, like magic, the top of the moon appeared over the ridgeline. It pushed up through the scrub – a glowing egg stretching higher, higher – then burst round and huge from the treetops. That has to be a sign.

10 February

There's always something to marvel over, if you're looking. I returned to the bush reserve today and saw a group of crested pigeons strolling through the grass beside the track, unperturbed by Chico on his lead. Finally we got too close and they all took off with that peculiar whistling beat of their wings. I'd always taken this noise for granted, but now I wanted to know more. So I went home and looked it up.

These pigeons have a modified primary flight feather that produces its distinctive noise. The beat is faster and more urgent when the bird takes off steeply, as it does when startled. Many pigeon and dove species do the same – signalling alarm to others with wingbeats described as a whistle, whirr, roar or frrr.

That's my nature fact for the day.

Now on to cancer facts.

My breast cancer has been treated, but the whole of me has not. I never anticipated the cancer chasm waiting for me when I hopped off Linac 2 for the last time. Until that point, I was well looked after, but once I walked out the door of the radiation oncology wing, I was pretty much on my own.

I suppose it has to be that way – the medical resources used to treat me were enormous, and no society can afford to mollycoddle someone once 'cured'. And I'm grateful, don't get me wrong. My experience of conventional cancer treatment has been excellent. I've found medical people to be friendly, informative and patient with my many enquiries. They seem genuinely concerned for my welfare, and believe in the effectiveness of their treatments.

And I've received great support along the way: home visits after surgery from nurses; sessions with breast care nurses and follow up support calls; information sessions for chemotherapy and radiotherapy treatments; and referrals for cancer counselling, physiotherapy and oncology massage.

I've had lovely experiences, too. People going out of their way to support cancer patients with no payment except the joy that comes with helping others. Here's a stand-out example.

One hot day soon after my hair fell out, I went to a shop selling headwear for people like me. I walked in all sweaty and grumpy, and hovered behind a hat stand feeling awkward. Then I was spotted by the volunteer staff.

Two women sat me down in front of a mirror, plied me with cold water and cups of tea, and modelled a range of exotic head coverings on my roughly shaved head. I laboured to copy their neat little twists and ties to produce glamorous do's that my belly-dancing friend (aka scarf-tying expert) would've been proud of. Other women came and went, unveiling their fluffy or shiny heads for decoration, and watching my modelling show with enthusiasm.

I walked out two hours later laden with gifts and pretty purchases, my spirits lifted by these generous women.

On another occasion, I went to a free session called 'Look Good – Feel Better', run by volunteers to help women with cancer manage the ugly side effects. We sat around a large table, some of us with wigs and headscarves, some fairly normal-looking, others frail – but all of us determined to enjoy ourselves. We plastered our pallid faces with donated make-up and laughed as the braver ones amongst us whipped off head covers and modelled various wigs. I made myself look macabre with clumsy use of an eyebrow pencil, and reassured myself that it didn't matter – I was in no danger of losing my eyebrows. (Wrong, as it turned out.)

Mind you, when it got to the point later on where I probably needed my little stash of donated make-up, I figured it was all too obvious what my affliction was to bother fussing. Here's the equation: middle-aged woman + rainbow headscarf + tired/lined face + sickly/gaunt appearance = CANCER. It's a no-brainer.

But back to my main point about cancer treatment. Despite the niceness of the mainstream cancer specialists I've dealt with, at the end of the day, their focus is always on my breasts, my lymph nodes and my 'system' (in case of metastasis). The whole of me, Kate the person, is of lower priority. They're not paid to assess me as an individual – to consider my lifestyle, my emotional state, or any but the most obvious health issues that may have led to me getting cancer.

And the other, more peripheral practitioners I saw while undergoing treatment – all of them helpful, caring people – had a necessarily limited focus as well. For example, I saw a specialist physiotherapist who helped me with the lymphatic cording in my surgery arm, but couldn't help me with the chemo-scarring in my left arm veins or the muscular problems brought on by radiotherapy. Another woman gave me delightfully soothing oncology massages and inadvertent counselling as we talked in a darkened room, but she had to refer me elsewhere for advice about my compressed neck vertebrae and hormonal therapy concerns. An osteopath did wonders for my neck and back problems, and gave me plenty of general advice, but she was wary of giving specific cancer-related advice because that wasn't her specialty.

It's all understandable. But what it adds up to is lots of people helping bits of me. In short, the only person it seems who can be holistic – who can work out what I need in the longer term – has to be…ta da! Me.

15 February

I'm back to thinking about my aura – the energy 'force field' surrounding me. If you want to feel it, try this.

Stand easily, shoulders relaxed, feet slightly apart. Breathe slowly, quiet your thoughts. Take a deep breath, lift your arms above your head until your palms touch (or close enough). Now breathe out slowly and start to lower your arms with your elbows slightly bent and your hands facing inwards, as if trying to feel the edges of an oval balloon surrounding you. As you're lowering your arms, gently draw them closer to your body and you should notice a point at which your hands start to tingle. Very gently, bring your hands closer and see if you notice a feeling of resistance that gets stronger as your hands approach your body. Then move your hands away again and feel the resistance decrease.

If you're like me, you'll find it soon becomes easy to sense the edges of the energy field enveloping you. And if you do it often enough, you'll notice that on days when you're tired, sad, run-down – that kind of thing – your energy field is smaller and weaker. But it can be strengthened.

Yesterday I was out walking, my mind busy so I wasn't really noticing the bush around me. But I knew I felt depleted. I was doing a few arm and shoulder exercises as I walked, which reminded me to check my aura. Sure enough, my energy field was thin (maybe only half an arm's length). I've a few ways of repairing this, but this time I wondered if a simple technique I described a while back was all I needed.

So I breathed in the good energy of the sky, trees and air above me and let it run down through me, then breathed it out through my feet and into the ground. Another breath to draw in the energy of the earth and let it stream up through me and out, pushing it into the skies. A couple of repetitions and already I felt lighter and easier.

Sure enough, another check revealed my aura to be much bigger. Just like that.

This isn't a miracle cure, rather a quick fix. Problems need more work than that to go away. But nonetheless, when my energy field is stronger, I feel better. It's that simple.

And here's something I just noticed. If I feel my aura while sitting, it's smaller and somehow bumpy. Telling, isn't it?

We spend way too much time sitting. Slumped over, breathing shallowly, focusing for hours on a computer or a TV or a book. Our attention is caught up in mind stuff while our bodies slowly fester.

The times in my life when I've felt most healthy are when I've been constantly up and about for long periods. Like when picking fruit for weeks over the summer holidays at home, or on field research trips during uni, or of course on bushwalks.

*

A friend of mine went bushwalking at Cradle Mountain in Tasmania recently. Before she left, she told me about the challenges of packing food, fuel and equipment for ten days. With no fires allowed and all waste having to be carried out, this was no small task. We laughed at the choices she faced: was bringing a novel more important than chocolate? If she took wine, should she share it with the friend who refused to bring any?

Which got me wondering…when did I last hoist my pack onto my shoulders and set off into wilderness?

I think it was at Mootwingie National Park on a three or four-day walk with my friend Tara. My memories are fuzzy but I know we found Aboriginal carvings and relics, climbed rocky outlooks and ate chocolate, and did a lot of sitting around the campfire drinking tea and port. And cooking old favourites liked stuffed pumpkin wrapped in foil and baked in the coals – not something you could take on a ten-day trip in Tassie, sadly. Yep, that was it. The very last backpacking trip.

But why do I keep returning to this theme? Do I really have a desperate need to take up hiking again? I'm older, spoilt, perhaps even a bit lazy. When I picture my friend in Tassie trudging along with her eighteen-kilogram pack, fighting the natural tendency to hunch over and watch the ground (to counterbalance the weight)…well, no, I'm honest enough to admit I never really enjoyed the actual *walking* part of such trips. What I loved was when I took my pack off and felt my whole body lifting up, almost floating without the weight. Then being able to sit in some glorious spot, drink thirstily and snack on something yummy. Everything tasted great on bushwalks. Even tea made with powdered milk, and dry biscuits spread with margarine. And I loved the evenings, when a level bank beside a creek bed could turn into a little village of tents clustered around a crackling fire.

I miss all that. And I miss the humble connection a long bushwalk gives you with your body. You can't ignore your physical needs (and limitations) when out bush for days. I can't imagine being able to get breast cancer if I went bushwalking every few months. Why? Because I'd notice during the walks if I'd lost my energy. Or if I'd gained weight, drunk too much wine, got too sad – the heaviness of it would slow me down. I'd know I was in trouble. And then – as the days of walking and good, simple food worked their magic – the heaviness would slough away and I'd be reminded of who I was. And what I needed to do to stay that way.

21 February

Damn, time's running through my fingers like sand – but is it red inland sand or bright beach sand? The former speaks of past times and old landscapes, the latter of movement and new life.

I'm back at my friend's coast house for the weekend, this time by myself. The sea is close, you can smell it, hear it, but there's thick scrub and swamp between us. It's nice to sit on the back deck overlooking the bush and watch the parade of life before me. Everywhere there's movement. Scrub turkeys strutting through the undergrowth, kangaroos preening themselves on the lawn next door, birds flitting in amongst low shrubs. And ants – they're everywhere! If you look closely, the grass below the deck is dense with their little sandy nests.

As dusk falls, fruit bats squabble and take flight from the tree canopy while mosquitoes emerge from cool hideaways for their evening onslaught. Inside, a baby huntsman spider splayed on the ceiling waits for me to turn off the lights before it goes on the prowl.

You couldn't live here and continue seeing yourself as somehow set apart from this verdancy of living. We're all part of the great cycle.

Earlier today, I walked with my dog on a track which runs behind the dunes lining the shore. Something heavier than usual went crashing through the undergrowth behind me and I turned to see Chico (the little bugger) hot on its heels. Then he stopped abruptly, ears drooping uncertainly as he considered his options. I trotted back to see what was going on, and there it was. A huge goanna halfway up a gum tree, gripping the smooth bark with strong claws. It must've been two and a half metres from head to tail.

'That's some lizard you've flushed out, Chico,' I said, amazed.

The goanna glared down at Chico and hissed loudly. Chico returned its gaze but with wilted bravado. Then he turned away.

I laughed. Goanna, 1; dog, 0.

22 February

Driving home from the coast today, I'd barely gone a kilometre when I had to stop to let a waddling echidna cross the road. I love echidnas. They're such funny, squat-looking creatures with their spines swaying as they move. This one was still ambling across the tarmac when a car appeared ahead of me. I stuck my arm out the window to warn the driver of my curious little companion, and he braked to avoid the echidna, then waved at me as he passed. We drove our separate ways, happy the echidna was safe.

Isn't it funny that we humans do this? Why go to all this trouble to protect an animal that we rarely interact with? I find that marvellous. You can find so much animal goodness around you, if you start looking.

Like Chico. He's parked himself on the carpet behind me as I type, and will lie there for hours, just content to be near me. It's true that I feed him and look after his needs – but nonetheless it's obvious he likes my company. Despite evolutionary advantage and ecological imperatives, at the end of the day my dog cares for me. When I'm crying, he nudges my hand and watches me soulfully. When I'm happy, his eyes brighten.

I love that we animals have this ability. To care, to love.

23 February

I'm done with seeing people in the hope they can quickly make me better. Truly.

A couple of weeks ago, I went to a traditional Chinese medicine (TCM) practitioner. I'd hoped he would give me a holistic assessment of where I'm at, maybe offer me some acupuncture to unblock my energy meridians and help with the compressed discs in my neck. At the very least, he could give me some miracle Chinese potion to restore my mojo.

No such luck. There's no magic bullet out there for me. When am I going to learn?

My TCM man directed me to lie fully clothed on a massage table, then held each of my wrists and felt my pulse as we talked about my health. Finally he declared that my system was surprisingly strong after what I'd been through, but only because I was strong before. Then came the clanger. Despite all that, my system was about as robust as a drug addict's. (Yes, he actually said that.)

Next he pushed firmly just beneath my ribs on the right side and declared my liver to be okay. Phew.

He said he could give me Chinese herbs to help strengthen my system, explaining that they're pretty much a form of high-potency nutrition which would give me a boost. I could achieve the same with diet, but it would take longer. And if I wanted the best results, I should try something like Qi Gong or Tai Chi, but it would take months before I'd really notice any improvements.

Finally he massaged my shoulders and neck to try release the tightness. He said he might be able to reposition the vertebrae so they weren't compressing the discs. The massage was firm and almost unpleasant, and at the end my skin was sore and red. I hoped this was a good thing.

Afterwards, I asked for details of the herbs he wanted to give me but he said it was a complicated mix and couldn't tell me. I explained that I was nervous about putting unknown substances in my body after having cancer, but that didn't persuade him. He said I didn't need to take them if I didn't want to.

I walked out stiff and sore, and a little deflated.

He wanted me to come back a week later so he could have another go at my neck and shoulders, and after much thought I returned. The herbs I would forgo, but the chance to make my neck better couldn't be missed.

This time, I got an even more vigorous massage culminating in an uncomfortable workout on my neck. It was hard to stay relaxed and I sighed with relief when he finished. But it seemed to help. After the stiffness wore off a few days later, I decided the numbness in my hands was fading, and was optimistic that each day would see an improvement.

But after my weekend at the coast, I came home with a stiff neck. Last night, I slept badly, changed pillows several times, tossed and turned and cursed. Most likely it was from the car drive, or from the cleaning up I did before leaving the house, but either way I was back to square one. Back to my cycle.

Feel better → start doing more → feel worse again → get sad.

No shortcuts for me. My weakened muscles and impoverished (drug addict) system need time.

2 March

There's usually a sign – a moment when I stop and look around, alerted to the approach of a new season. Yesterday it was the late afternoon light on the local oval: a yellowish light, picking out the greens of the grass and trees with a peculiar intensity. Telling me that autumn is coming.

I know most people see spring as a time of newness and growth, but for me I think that time is autumn. When the days are shortening and the trees closing down production for the winter – that's when I come alive. I love the crackle of cold in the morning air and the way everything sounds different. The calling of cockatoos echoes further, people's voices are clearer as they walk nearby, car traffic is more intense. And while I haven't noticed that change in sound yet, just the light, it will come. A moment when I pause, listening, and then sigh happily.

It brings my thoughts to cold weather pastimes. Long walks in the midday sun, trips to the coast where the sea rushes coldly up the sand and each breath shocks the lungs. And skiing, oh yeah.

Last year, we went downhill skiing for a day late in the season. It was my birthday – forty-eight, woo hoo! Not likely. I was depressed from Tamoxifen and still recovering from radiotherapy. Not much to celebrate. But I managed the skiing okay so that made me happy. For a day, I could shake off the shackles of cancer treatment and forget my normal life. Catch a lift, admire the snow-laden trees, the blue-white snow banks hidden in shadows, the beady eyes of a crow watching the passing parade. Focus on the basics: exercise, warmth, food, self-protection.

That's one thing I love about such extreme environments. Even though we pretend that we've tamed the ski slopes, it only needs a day of sleet and icy winds to remind us that life is tenuous. Despite the parade of trendy outfits and the casual chatter of people drinking hot chocolates behind foggy windows, outside the world is harsh. Real.

I love it all. The clanking of the heavy machinery running the lifts, the wet cold of the metal chairlifts, the bone-chilling wetness that creeps through cheap snow gear as the first flurry of snow flakes turn to soggy sleet.

Bring it on.

3 March

While at uni, I went on a week-long cross-country skiing trip. It still amazes me that we got off so lightly, given our inexperience. So much could have gone wrong. But that's what being young is about, isn't it? Doing rather than thinking.

We started our expedition at Falls Creek, stomping past brightly clothed downhill skiers in our motley assortment of clothes cobbled together from friends, family and op shops. I wore itchy woollen pants from an army disposals store, layers of itchy woollen jumpers, itchy overpriced new woollen socks, and non-itchy synthetic gloves and balaclava through which the cold was already trickling. My newly waterproofed japara barely fit over the top of all my layers.

Yep, I was comfy all right.

Then we hired our skis – old-style ones that clipped onto our own boots, which in my case were Blundstones with stiff leather and worn soles. The experienced guys in our group demonstrated the parallel sliding technique needed to propel ourselves along the flat ground and we mucked around for a bit trying it out. So far, so good.

But when we hauled our loaded packs onto our backs, the equation changed. To counteract the weight, you have to lean forward a bit more, but this makes it hard to glide forward smoothly on the skis. Lean back a little to change the weight distribution and you can guess what happens. Over backwards, legs kicking like an upturned beetle.

I'd been to the snowfields once during primary school but had only tobogganed. This was new to me. So it was enough of a struggle staying upright to even notice that one ski wasn't clipping to my boot very well, making it wobble and splay to the side as I pushed it forwards.

Time was slipping away and soon we had to head off. Our destination was an alpine hut a few kilometres away – just a tiny distance really, we'd be there in a snap.

It took hours. I'd mastered skiing on flat ground (sort of), but in undulating terrain, oh my. Going downhill, the idea is to bend your knees, let your skis run in the tracks of the person in front and just go. Whee! Or not. My tendency was to panic as I got faster, straighten up to slow myself, lose my balance and fall over backwards. (Refer to beetle comment above.) Or if I was going too fast, I'd turn my skis, plough through softer snow and end up face-first with my pack pinning me down.

As for going uphill…if you've tried skiing, you'll know how hard that is. (Picture a spider trying to climb out of a bathtub and you won't be far off.)

Finally we got to the hut, dumped our packs and collapsed. Time for the best cup of tea ever.

But here's something we hadn't considered. Getting water in the snowfields should be easy (we'd thought about that) and below the hut was a creek that was frozen over but still flowing. We could either crack through the ice, or if lazy simply collect a saucepan of snow from near the hut and melt it over the stove. We chose the latter.

This was a hut used frequently in the winter. Some campers slept inside, others set up tents around it. There was a pit toilet down the hill, but in the dark of night some took easier options. And as for food scraps and cooking waste – some buried or burnt them, others scuffed snow over them or, worse, chucked them under a tree when no one was looking.

My point? Alpine huts, back then at least, were a hygiene nightmare.

So we had our tea and a snack, mucked around on our skis for a bit (so much easier without a pack on) and then set up for dinner. No doubt it was macaroni cheese, I don't remember, but I do remember the port and chocolate Tim Tams that followed because soon after Tony hightailed it outside and threw up in the snow. We lamented the loss of the port and biscuits, and joked about him being a cheap drunk as he sloped off to his hard bunk.

All very funny until the early hours of the morning when I woke with my guts churning. Uh oh. I barely had time to grab the garbage bag I'd set aside for wet clothes before throwing up all my Tim Tams and port into it. Five minutes later, I was stumbling through the snow to the pit toilet with my baggie of vomit and a torch. I tipped the contents down the hole, got a whiff of the smell rising from the long drop, then promptly emptied into it whatever was left in my guts.

I was okay the next day, but over the week as we moved from hut to hut, all but one of us got sick. Never have I been on a trip where we brought so much food and ate so little. Oh, the joys.

And we were lucky. The weather was kind to us. Each evening, we attempted to dry our soggy, stinky clothes but this wasn't much of a problem because the days were sunny and benign. We were often cold but never dangerously so. Nobody got injured, or disappeared in a white-out. It took me a day or so to work out that my ski boot clips were faulty, and by then I couldn't do anything about it. Falling over and skiing badly was my lot for the week, along with the sore knee I developed from constantly correcting the wayward ski. But I was fit and strong, so I got by. And because we stayed in huts, whoever was sick at the time had somewhere to lie around groaning and a toilet to run to.

It occurred to me afterwards that things could've gone awry very quickly, but hey, I was young. These things happened to other people, not me.

And here's what I took away with me. Away from the crowds, the high country in winter is breathtaking. The creamy-barked snow gums are achingly beautiful against a patchwork of intense blue sky. In the stillness, the landscape feels vast and ancient. I still remember skiing past a smoothly curving snow bank in the shadows, and feeling its icy blueness cut straight to my soul.

And the silence – insulated by snow and cold – there's nothing like it.

Oh yeah, do it.

5 March

It's nice disappearing into my past, because reality ain't so easy.

Yesterday, I went for a routine check-up with my radiation oncologist. She listened to my heart and lungs, then palpated my depleted breasts – all the time chatting away. I wasn't quite so calm. What was she listening for in my heart and lungs? Can you detect cancer like that? And my breasts, well…not much happening there but perhaps she'd find something I hadn't?

But no, all good. With a sigh, I sat down for a check-up chat.

First we discussed the breast scans I'd had a few months before. As far as I was concerned, I had nothing to worry about – that's what my oncologist had said when he saw the results – but my radiologist wasn't so sure.

The lymph node they'd commented on, according to her, was slightly enlarged. This was news to me – I'd been given the impression they weren't absolutely sure it was a lymph node, hence the need for another 'routine' scan in six months (rather than the usual twelve).

But no, she explained that the problem was the size of the node. Ah…now I got it. Of course enlarged lymph nodes are quite normal in most cases. We all know that feeling of sore glands in our neck when we've got a cold – busy lymph nodes are bigger lymph nodes. But for someone like me, a busy lymph node in my breast could be bad news.

She assured me that it's likely nothing to worry about and the next scan will probably show a normal-sized lymph node again. Hmm, tell that to my panicking brain.

What amazes me about the medical system is how ad hoc it can be. Why wasn't I told this earlier? Even with all the technology at hand, the advice I get depends on who I talk to and what questions I ask. And it's getting even harder now as I cycle through quarterly check-ups with my three specialist doctors – all of whom communicate with each other but not as comprehensively as I'd like. They don't have time, and I'm not a priority case any more.

Here's more news from the medical profession. I told my radiologist that my breast still hurts when I run, and asked if that's normal. Yes, indeed. In fact, she said the pain may be coming from the ribs and tissue beneath my breast, still likely to be inflamed eight months after my treatment. Wow.

I know I shouldn't complain, but it's hard not knowing the full implications of what you're doing. But would I have done things differently if I'd known how many flow-on effects there'd be?

The trouble is, such information is always presented as a possibility. 'These are the sort of side effects you may have, but not everyone gets them.' That is, don't worry about it until you have to; all may be well. Yah de yah. I wonder how many people with cancer are worn down by a growing assortment of 'possible' side effects like mine. Most?

Here's the truth: if you have breast cancer treatment, you may not suffer from any one side effect, but you *will* suffer from many side effects – some of which may stay with you for years. Take it or leave it.

One spot of good news. When my radiologist asked the question I'd been dreading – had I started taking aromatase inhibitors – her response was surprisingly sympathetic. She said I'm obviously sensitive to these sorts of drugs and she understands my choice not to take them. Of course she said to consider taking them further down the track, 'when you feel more on top of things', but I know that ain't gonna happen.

Next we moved onto discussing my right hand, which was getting sore and slightly puffy when I did too many domestics (sweeping floors, vacuuming, pruning, mowing – lots of things actually). While I knew this might be a sign of lymphoedema, I'd convinced myself I wouldn't get that.

Lymphoedema is a potentially serious condition which can occur after the removal of lymph nodes, as is commonly done during cancer surgeries. Lymph nodes and lymph vessels form a network which removes cell debris and foreign bodies like bacteria (and cancer cells) from body tissue and returns them to the blood system. When lymph nodes are removed, this puts stress on the local lymph vessels and makes it harder for them to channel fluid back to the heart. If fluid starts accumulating in body tissue and isn't removed, further complications arise. Women who develop advanced lymphoedema after breast cancer surgery may end up with a permanently swollen arm (or arms) and recurrent, debilitating infections. Once diagnosed, the usual treatment is to wear a compression sleeve 24/7, at least to begin with, and avoid situations which bring on swelling.

You'd think the problems I had with cording of my lymph vessels after surgery would've rung a few alarm bells, but no. I continued telling myself I was slim and active – of course I wouldn't get lymphoedema. Sound familiar?

My radiologist wasted no time putting me straight. It was clear I was suffering symptoms of mild lymphoedema – which incidentally is more common than people think. (Excuse me, why hadn't anyone told me this either?)

Another strike.

But to my surprise she said not to worry: it wasn't necessarily a sign I was going to end up wearing a compression sleeve. It just meant I would have to be more careful, and try to avoid or do less of the activities that cause the puffiness and pain.

So, not as bad as I imagined but…it's one more flow-on effect I hadn't anticipated.

Here comes the recurring theme. 'Why me?'

13 March

Last weekend, I went on a short bushwalk with a friend. Well, 'short' was the plan.

It was a great morning with blue skies and crisp air. Where I live you can go to any number of wild places within an hour's drive, so by 9.30 we were on the trail to Square Rock. In just under an hour's walk, we made it to our rocky eyrie, and stood looking out over mountains and fire-scarred scrub.

The bushland around my home is full of spots like this one – high ridges or peaks capped with jumbled granite boulders. Square Rock is a whopper – a two-tiered lump of rock perched on a motley selection of haphazardly arranged boulders. One day, Square Rock is going to teeter and fall with an almighty crash into the deep valley below.

But it sat there for us, docile in the sunshine – a quiet haven for skinks, ants and us. We drank tea, ate banana bread and surveyed the sweeping valley and hills before us. What could be better for the soul?

Eventually, people started arriving – it was a public holiday and a perfect autumn day, after all – so we packed up and headed back.

So far, so good. Despite my relative lack of fitness I felt great, so my friend talked me into taking a longer route home. All fine, except it turned out to be further than we'd anticipated. Plus it was getting hot, with long sections of the walk in full sunshine. As we plodded along, my feet began to drag and my back ache. So much for feeling great.

Halfway along, we found a little creek full of icy-cold water and sat for a while, staving off the hot track ahead of us. It was peaceful watching the tiny fish and water beetles doing their thing, listening to the soft gurgle of mountain water. I felt a bit better, but not for long.

On with our packs and into the sunshine. Plod plod, grit teeth, try to chat nicely, grit teeth, stomp stomp. Sigh.

I ran out of puff. My back muscles seized up and my scarred underarm ached badly from where my daypack straps were rubbing. I had no reserves. Nothing.

Of course I got by. My friend took my (not very heavy) daypack and despite my slowing progress we still found lots to look at and enjoy.

But it made me sad. Are my thoughts of doing an overnight walk before winter overambitious? I'm so damaged. So tentative. Like one of those water beetles in the creek – skating along the surface, diving down every now and then but quickly rising back up.

17 March

My eldest daughter has booked her trip to Europe. She's going by herself, so it's a big deal. I can't imagine doing such a thing at her age and it makes me terribly anxious, wondering how she'll manage.

Ah, the cycle of life. I went to India on my own in my early twenties and hardly spared a thought for my worried parents. After all, I was a grown-up. An independent woman! Why fuss?

My parents had a good reason for not wanting me to go – but unfortunately it was the very same reason motivating me to leave. Life back then was way too overwhelming, and I had to run away. So six months after Michael's death, I vanished too.

It's a funny thing, travelling. It brings out the best in me. I'm resourceful, curious and full of energy – so perfectly able to look after myself. In India, I was more assertive. I could bat off men's approaches with ease, speak my mind nicely but firmly, and radiate a confidence that kept me safe. How was it that as soon as I returned home with my new strength, it began draining away?

18 March

Can I go back to India and find that girl again?

Several years ago, no doubt with similar thoughts in mind, I started writing a story based on my trip. Here are a few pages, so you can see where it's leading me.

*

To my surprise, the rickshaw driver, who'd shown no sign of understanding me, dropped me right outside the YMCA. He only charged twice what the Guide predicted. I found a large armchair in the lobby and collapsed. Barely nine a.m. and I was shattered.

After a few minutes, I approached the reception desk.

'No, madam, we have no single rooms, only double.'

'Are you sure?'

The plump woman in peacock blue simply tilted her head in a gesture I would see many times. It seemed to mean 'what more can be said?'

I turned away, unbelieving. Then picked up my pack, expecting the woman to call, 'Madam, there has been a mistake, we have a room!' People back home had warned me of this: expect trickery, be vigilant. Everyone wants your money in India!

But the woman said nothing. I could turn round, take the double room, pay four times what I'd been hoping to pay. But now, mortifyingly, my eyes were filling with tears. I wasn't cut out for this.

Back in the armchair, I gazed unseeingly at my Guide. Tucked in the middle was my boyfriend's photo, taken in his front yard on a sunny day. It wasn't such a good photo – his face was half in shadow, and he stood self-consciously. My tears dripped onto the page beside it.

No. I shut the book and wiped my eyes. This was pathetic.

And now a German voice caught my attention. A tall, confident-looking girl asking for a room. Again came the line about no singles, but this girl didn't argue. She took the double. As she turned away, key in hand, I jumped up.

'Hi, I'm looking for a room too. Maybe we can share?'

Had I really done that? But the girl spoke English, she was a lifeline and I grabbed hold.

*

The German girl's name was Kirsten. She was just back from the mountains, a place called Leh, and was desperate for some fresh fruit. Would I like to go with her to buy some? I nodded, grateful. If it was just me, I'd have stayed in this clean, quiet room all day.

Kirsten laid a sheet out on her bed and eyed my bare mattress. 'They don't always supply sheets. You know that, don't you?'

'Oh.'

'Don't worry – we'll fix that. We're in India. Everything's cheap!'

*

With Kirsten at my side, Delhi was transformed. I copied my new friend's purposeful stride and 'don't mess with me' gaze. The trick seemed to be to let your eyes slide over people's faces without engaging with them. No expression, no acknowledgement – at least not until ready. This worked a charm: people watched but didn't approach.

The sidewalks were filling up now. I gasped at a sheet spread on the stained concrete covered with a gorgeous array of spices: each in a perfect conical pile. A wrinkled old woman brandished a tiny cup made from newspaper, grinning widely through her one, blackened tooth. Beside her was a battered cart selling fresh sugar cane juice, then a brazier topped with charred corn which smelt like heaven. Up ahead was a long line of fruit vendors, heralded by a cart offering beautifully carved pineapple segments set in ice.

I remembered I hadn't had breakfast.

'It's a public holiday,' said Kirsten, 'that's why the streets are so quiet.'

'They are?' I eyed the cars and motorbikes rushing past, trying to imagine what 'busy' must be like. Then turned back just in time to avoid stepping on a freshly laid cowpat, the owner of which was nearby, grazing on discarded sugar cane leaves.

'The cows do whatever they want here,' laughed Kirsten. 'So watch your step.'

I glanced at her flimsy sandals and cringed, imagining the disease and filth she must be exposing herself to. But my own sensible sandshoes were making my feet itchy and hot.

'Let's get a pineapple juice,' said Kirsten.

'But what about bugs in the water?'

'It's just juice, and they peel the pineapple first – don't worry about it.'

But I ended up with a 'safe' bottle of cola while Kirsten drained her golden juice with a sigh of pleasure. The cola was barely cold, not that I could complain for one rupee.

The man selling it yelled at me as I made to leave, gesturing at a row of empty bottles. Ah, recycling at its best, I thought, stopping and finishing my drink. A cluster of men stood around drinking theirs – all watching me, of course. But when I returned the bottle, the vendor flashed me a smile and I smiled back.

*

I surprised myself by spending several hours without thinking of him.

We were served dhal and rice in a cramped restaurant beneath rickety *fans. The tables and chairs were plastic, the plates and cutlery the thinnest of metal. Kirsten gulped down the water served in smudged aluminium cups, I asked for a bottle.*

'It's freshly cooked,' stated Kirsten, gesturing to the giant pot of dhal on the boil nearby.

I wondered how she could be so sure, but my stomach was rumbling. We'd washed our hands at a basin in a dark corner, but even so I hesitated to pick up the warm chapati from the plate beside me.

Kirsten dipped one in dhal and bit into it, grinning as the lentils dripped between her fingers. 'It's good!'

And it was – wondrously good. I ate ravenously, scooping up mouthfuls of perfectly cooked rice and aromatic, oily dhal. Suddenly this grimy place full of foreign people felt cosy and benign.

The feeling faded quickly as we walked out into the street. The air was hot and thick, and the sidewalks jammed with people. I paused to watch a woman with red-stained teeth carefully placing an assortment of spices and dried substances onto a leaf, then rolling it up with deft fingers. She handed it to the man in front of her, who stuffed the bundle in his mouth and chewed vigorously.

'It's called paan,' said Kirsten, enjoying my astonishment. 'Betel leaf with some kind of palm nut and tobacco and spices inside – it gives you a nice buzz. You should try it.'

I eyed the man, still chewing, as he wiped a dribble of red from his stained mouth. 'Um, another time.'

My eyes strayed to a row of beggars on the ground. A girl with a stump for an arm looked up at me and I stared back, stricken. Then I jumped back hastily as the man from the paan stand spat a great mouthful of red juices on the pavement.

'You've got to see this.' Kirsten grabbed my hand and tugged me towards some stairs leading down into darkness.

Stuffy air rose to meet us but I didn't mind. Better that than those beggars, and that man, spattering us with his disdain.

It was an underground market. Narrow tunnels ran in concentric circles, lined with rows of tiny shops. Many were closed for the holiday, but even so it was overwhelming. I followed close on Kirsten's heels, trying to stay within my new friend's forcefield of confidence. Nonetheless hands reached out, 'Come, come', and voices chased after me, 'Special price, first customer!' They acted as if my acquiescence was a done deal, as if I'd agreed to go with them before they even spoke.

My lesson for the day seemed to be to look without looking, to absorb this new world while appearing to ignore it. I was an actor in a play I didn't understand. But soon the magic of shopping worked its charm, and I found myself agreeing to meet Kirsten at the same spot in an hour. Once alone, oddly, I felt free. The game was getting easier, and somehow I was starting to enjoy myself. The purchase of a pair of camel-hide shoes with curling pointed toes earned me a cup of sweet tea. My lengthy exclamations over a rack of silky, baggy pants brought out shy giggles from a young woman with a sparkling nose-piercing. Four men lined up to help me try on some pretty leather sandals with gold braid across the top, clapping as I tossed my sweaty sandshoes into a flimsy plastic bag and walked out with the cool sandals on my feet.

Hours later, Kirsten and I emerged like wraiths, blinking in the late afternoon sun.

Kirsten linked her arm through mine. 'Let's go get a cup of tea.'

*

As we sat at a table beside a potted palm, I remembered. My man, left behind. I wondered if he'd felt the absence of my thoughts, and was ashamed. He'd be working, living a normal day, and here I was being served tea from a heavy silver pot by a waiter with a white napkin draped across one arm. I almost laughed aloud, picturing how I must look. But then the familiar heaviness swooped down on me. I was so far away. What was I doing?

*

India had a definite smell. I inhaled quietly, trying to find the source. It was there, beneath the chemical tang of my new sleeping sheet; it was *caught in the stuffing of my lumpy pillow. It was everywhere, at the airport, on the bus, on the streets of Delhi, and now here, in the quiet of night.*

Dust, incense, concrete, deprivation... I heard the clang of metal on metal, and the laughter of children. Outside, India was still busy.

What time would it be back home? He'd be eating dinner, or maybe out at a pub with friends. Was he thinking of me? I tried to picture him, but all I got was the awkward shadowy face from my photo. As I drifted off to sleep, another photo appeared in my mind. A teenage boy in a sleeping bag, smiling sheepishly as the camera caught him mid-wriggle, trying to change his underwear.

Now I was there, kneeling beside him. I could smell the bush around us, the woodsmoke from our breakfast fire. 'I'm sorry,' I said. 'I'm sorry. I shouldn't have yelled at you when you were overtaking that truck on the way here. It was my fault we almost crashed.'

But as I spoke his smile dissolved, and the sleeping bag fell empty to the ground.

I jerked awake to the smell of smoke, of someone cooking dinner on an old kerosene stove.

20 March

That girl who went to India on her own isn't as far from me as I thought. Now I can see that I wasn't so much brave as determined. I needed to prove something to myself: that my life wasn't confined by the terrible event I'd just lived through.

Death and grief shadowed me, but despite my sadness I chose to look outwards and forwards. In India, I learned that I could look after myself – that I'd be okay, in time.

Strength is a relative thing. It comes and goes. Sometimes it's there when we need it, sometimes not. But when we're down, others can share their strength with us.

Back then, I thought that looking after myself meant doing it alone. Now I know that's not always possible. And more than that, now I know I don't need to do it alone.

21 March

That photo of Mike in my story was taken early one morning during a walk in the Flinders Ranges. I'd snapped him kneeling inside his sleeping bag putting on his jocks, so here was another situation where I'd managed to embarrass him. At the time, I thought nothing of it – isn't that what siblings do: invade each other's personal space and laugh about it? But many times since, I've looked at that photo and wondered if the grin on his face was closer to a grimace. Was he merely embarrassed or was he already deeply sad? I'll never know. But I don't think it was me who made him sad. An annoying sister fussing over him and treating him like a kid brother in front of her friends? Not so terrible.

I'm glad I keep thinking of him. Many people would say it's good because I need to 'let go'. That the trauma of his death may still be eating away at me and that I need to 'deal with it'. Sounds so trite to me. But there may be some truth in it. Over the years, I've dealt with the trauma by tidying Mike away in some neat corner of my mind, only letting him out when suits. That's no way to manage death, is it? It's time to carry him along openly in my heart.

24 March

It's been a while since I've visualised my energy colours, so today I had a go – hoping for some nice green and orange instead of the usual murkiness.

Except I couldn't 'see' colours at all. Rather, I felt my energy as relative density. My abdomen and legs were okay, fairly light, but my chest, back and neck area were a different story. That hump on my back? Still there, but now spreading into a dense ball of black weightiness, an energy basketball in my upper torso. So much for progress.

So I started breathing into the ball, filling it with the world's good energy. And I know you'll think 'she's going off again', but I swear I felt an unfurling. My shoulder blades, all pointy and stressed and sad, began to release. I wriggled them as if shaking them out and they formed beautiful, strong wings. Broad, snow-white wings like

Pegasus's. The blackness from the ball drained out along the wings and became grey and then white.

At that point, I remembered a dream my twin brother had a few years after Michael died. He was sleeping in his room in the top loft – the one next to Michael's room – and he felt himself lifting from the bed and being pulled towards the wardrobe near the window. He passed through the clothes and the wall, and next was flying above the driveway and away into the night. The moon was out; he could see this peaceful, sleeping world beneath him. It was wonderful but also scary. He wondered if he'd ever go back to his body.

When Marty woke up, the image of that beautiful night-time world stayed with him – so much so that when he described it to me, I felt as if I'd dreamt it too.

As I lay there thinking about Marty's dream, the wings I'd been visualising lifted me up and their strength flowed into me. Not a transformation, rather a glimpse of what was on offer. I wondered if the person flying through the night was Michael. Had he given Marty his dream, and offered him his wings? And was he doing the same to me now?

13 April

Today while reading a book, I felt a welling up of knowledge. It goes like this.

I've been defined by fear – the fear of bad things happening. I learned way too early that things don't always work out for the best – that terrible things do happen. And for a dreamy girl who used to wander around her orchard home with a head full of made-up stories and adventures, this knowledge was heavy beyond belief.

I dealt with it by being stoic. Flattening my expectations. Getting on with things, hoping that in time all would be well again. And so it was, more or less. Except for the fear that dogged me, making me sidestep my way though life.

What doesn't kill you makes you stronger. That's the saying, but is it true? Coping is not the same as being stronger. My stoicism has protected me, but has also stopped me from experiencing the best that life offers.

As the character in the book I'm reading (*The White Mary* by Kira Salak) decides,

> ...no matter what tragedies in her life, no matter what horrors in the world...she must choose happiness for herself. She must. Or else the pain was all for nothing.

14 April

I went for a walk yesterday when the day was fading.

As I strode up a fire trail, busy with my thoughts, something made me stop and turn round. And there was the sun – glowing brilliant orange and huge. It was dropping from the clouds into a strip of clear sky above the mountain ranges. By some optical illusion, as I watched, the sun appeared to split in two: the top half still partly shaded by cloud, the bottom a brilliant half-orb bulging downwards into the clear sky as if being born. It felt like a sign. Of what, I'm not sure.

After a few minutes, the sun was gone behind the mountains and I kept on up the fire trail. But now my eyes found a shape on the hillside across from me. A fallen tree. The base of the tree appeared to rise up the hill like a head, the grey trunk curved sinuously towards me like a tail. It was a goanna, no doubt about it. The funny thing was that the tree had clearly fallen long before and I'd walked that way many times without noticing it.

You can look for signs everywhere, hmm? But still...

17 April

I had another ultrasound scan today.

As I lay on the bed with the probe passing over my skin, there was no way to avoid my fear. It's all so decisive – the clicking of the mouse, the tapping of keys, the insistent beeping as photo after photo is taken.

When I craned over my shoulder, I could just see the computer screen, enough to notice the dark nodules that the ultrasound technician kept zoning in on. These were the lymph nodes that had showed up in my scan late last year. Were they smaller than before? Or bigger? My racing pulse told me the latter.

The technician hurried out of the room to consult with the doctor, then returned saying she 'just needed a few more pictures of the right side'. As she started clicking and tapping away again, I lay paralysed. Convinced that this was it. I was heading for cancer land again.

I stayed silent as she worked, then wiped the slimy gel off my skin when she asked me to. Finally I sat up, pulled my hospital gown over me and gathered courage. 'Are those lymph nodes still enlarged?'

'Oh no,' she said brightly. 'They're normal, tiny actually. Nothing to worry about!'

OMG.

I drove home, dazed but smiling. And I'm still smiling.

29 April

Slowly but surely I feel it. The healing. It's been ten months since my last radiotherapy treatment, and nearly five months since finishing Tamoxifen – and now at last I can feel my strength returning.

Not every day. Yesterday I was tired, emotional and mentally dull – and cranked out my usual 'woe is me' routine. But today I'm much better.

Last week, I made it all the way up Mount Tennant (1,400 metres) with a friend; not bad for an old chook. Even though my energy bottomed within the first hour, I kept going and we made it to the top in three hours, and down in two and a half. Admittedly afterwards I had no energy for days, and even now my legs are a little stiff, but hey – it's an improvement.

And just when I thought my fingers would be numb forever, I find hours passing with nothing. Even at night I don't wake as often to assume the 'position' – flat on my back, hands by my side, no pillow.

Yep, I'm getting there.

12 May

Up and down, round and round – it's making me a little crazy. Chemo brain has descended upon me again. A smothering cloak of blurgh, turning me into this vague, emotional creature. I hate it.

This is my lot whenever I get stressed or tired. As I keep discovering, the improvements in my physical and mental state are tenuous. But this time I've crashed further. Why?

My daughter left for Europe last week. In the days before she left, I went on an overprotective mothering bender – writing lists, sorting bank cards and sim cards and travel insurance, buying bits and pieces – so many details, so much to remember! I stayed up late, fretting, adding to my lists. Then woke up at five a.m. fretting, adding to my lists. No doubt she couldn't wait to hop on that plane and get away from me.

After she left, I went to visit my folks for a few days – a distraction of sorts but no less stressful. When I see my parents, I end up torn between spending time with them, and spending time helping them (shopping, cleaning, cooking, organising). I rush around, busy busy busy. And when I stop, I feel intensely sad. Life contracts when you get to eighty-six, days are defined by medications, visits to doctors, staying warm, waiting for others to arrive. There's nothing fair about old age. What good am I, blowing in and helping for a few days then buggering off?

Now I'm home again, worn down. I feel the fog squeezing into my grey matter, robbing me of my memory and vitality. Not much stays in my head, even important things. My sentences come out all wrong, and reading the newspaper is a joke. (What's the issue again, who is this person?). I'm functioning – it's still me – but I feel like half of me. Give me a nudge and I'll collapse in a heap.

Argh!

16 May

Yesterday was the first frost. I ran outside when I saw the white sheen on the lawn and did a little dance on the frozen grass.

I've always loved frosty mornings. As a kid, I remember standing on our balcony and looking out over a world cloaked in ice. Denuded apple tree branches and grass fronds shining white as the sun rose. Veils of mist rising through the cold air. I loved puffing my warm breath out into the world – a reminder that I, too, was a part of things.

Weather like this makes me feel more alive. The world grabs me and shakes me – no hiding away inside my head.

But yesterday, even if I wanted to, there was no hiding. I went to a friend's house for coffee, walking through the cold air with the pompom on my beanie bouncing with my strides. Despite being in the doldrums only three days before, already I was on the up again.

My friend, however, wasn't so chirpy. She's had breast cancer too, although her story's different to mine. Her mastectomy went smoothly, and unlike me she didn't need chemotherapy, radiotherapy or hormone therapy. After a terrible start, things were looking good for her. That's until things stopped going according to plan.

Here it comes, the point at which the medical system raises its hands and says, 'What the?'

She'd been given a temporary breast implant during surgery, and for a while all was fine. Then she developed a seroma in her breast (it started filling with fluid), and she was told, 'These things happen. It'll pass.' But it didn't. Her breast became rock-hard and painful, but an ultrasound revealed only a small amount of fluid. She argued with the radiologist, who finally agreed to aspirate (stick a needle in and suck out the fluid). He removed 170 millilitres – a surprise to him but not her. After a short while, the fluid returned. She had it aspirated again, but this time the radiologist accidentally punctured the liquid-filled implant in her breast. Over the next few days, the implant emptied its contents into the surrounding tissue, leaving her with a deflated breast ('like a prune', she said) and a bubble of fluid collecting below her armpit. It took weeks of being shunted around before anything was done about it.

A week ago, she finally had surgery to replace the implant, and haemorrhaged during the operation. After a couple of days, she was sent home despite being in more pain than after her first surgery. A day or so later, she felt so unwell her eighty-seven-year-old mother drove her to casualty, and she was whisked off for emergency surgery with another haemorrhage. Nobody could say why it had happened – it was an 'extremely rare occurrence', which was no consolation for her.

When I saw her yesterday, she was home again, still in pain, and struggling with a surgery drain that was clogging up. But she doesn't want it removed yet – after all, there are no guarantees that once the drain is out her breast won't start filling with excess fluid again. And in a few months, when she gets a permanent implant, the whole ugly cycle could continue. (No surprise, as it turns out, that wasn't the end of the story. Three months later, she had surgery to put in a permanent implant and have her other breast lifted and reduced in size to match. Afterwards she developed a raging infection and was on antibiotics for weeks. This affected her 'normal' breast, which took ages to heal and developed keloid scarring. Now this breast has a thick, crumpled scar running from the base to the aureole, and the nipple is slightly disfigured. Throughout all this, she has stayed surprisingly positive. She's amazing.)

Even if there was a definitive manual for the expected after-effects of surgery, when it comes to the unexpected ones the manual is thrown in the recycling. The reassurances are thin, and the explanations vague.

I don't have answers for my friend either. All I can do is hug her and hope.

It reminds me that the less intervention you can get away with, the better. Do I really want to have my breast cut into again, just to make it look better? It's an option I'm considering, but is my vanity worth it? It's incredible what modern medicine can do, but doctors aren't demigods – they don't know everything. It's foolish to believe they can fix us like mechanics fix cars.

In a situation like breast cancer, which is often symptomless, it's easy to complain about the complications of treatment. I've been doing my fair share of that; it's hard not to. The treatment is brutal, with long-lasting and sometimes permanent side effects. But it's the best on offer, in a world awash with conflicting and confronting information. I chose to go with it, and here I am.

26 May

In our fish tank, we have three fish, hanging in there despite haphazard care and attention. Like all fish, they have a hierarchy: at the top is a pale yellow guppy who roams the tank keeping the other two in line; in the middle is a glowlight tetra who, despite being the smallest fish, manages to avoid much harassment; and at the bottom is Hope.

Hope is a survivor. When every adult platy in the aquarium died from a disease brought in on a new aquatic plant, baby Hope clung to life. We couldn't believe it when we spotted her – only a few millimetres long, swimming perkily around the empty tank. That was years ago, so she must be pretty old now.

Since then, we've kept other types of fish, most of whom have died, but Hope just keeps on keeping on. A few months ago, she developed a growth on her belly and her lopsided swimming convinced us she hadn't long for this earth. Not so. Despite ongoing bullying by Top Dog Guppy, her growth has disappeared and her swimming has improved.

She still hangs around near the bottom, making brief forays into open waters for food then diving down again, but somehow she's okay. In an ideal world, Hope should now be top dog. But life's not ideal. And despite the odds, Hope has managed to hang in there and make do.

There's a nice analogy for us all.

27 May

I took Chico for a walk in the dusk last night, my boots rudely loud on the footpath beside the soft clicking of doggy toenails. When we got to the park, Chico hauled on the lead as I struggled to unclip him, then hotfooted it to a tree nearby. As I approached, a bulky shadow high in the leafless branches gained shape: a fat brush-tail possum, its eyes just a glimmer in the darkness. Chico leapt and barked, scrabbled at the base of the trunk, then ran around in circles under the possum's calm gaze.

We kept walking and now I spotted a family of shadows: kangaroos, sitting motionless. Their silhouettes were unmistakable and comical – tiny heads perched on narrow shoulders over plump torsos. As we approached, they rose onto their powerful hind legs and bounded away – the adults unhurried and graceful, the joeys hesitant, turning to watch us then careening after their mums.

In the massive old gum behind me, a pair of sulphur-crested cockatoos were settling in for the night, their soft squeaks and gravelly squawks unmistakably personal – a dialogue of contented companionship.

As we neared home, a shadow slipped from our front yard onto the road – a neighbour's cat, checking things out while the coast was clear. Luckily, Chico didn't see or he'd have gone mental. Cats in his front yard – no way!

The outside light shone over our front deck and the rumble of the ducted heating invited me in, but I stood in the shadows for a few minutes watching this world around me. My home, so inviting and warm, is also a cage. The cars rushing past with their shadowy occupants and blinking lights? More cages.

As night falls and we humans scurry for cover, other animals emerge. What do they think of us hiding away in our muted bubbles?

I find it heartening that despite the mess we've made of things, animals are still surrounding us, adjusting, making do. Snacking on the plant bounty in our backyards, chatting in treetops, quietly grazing the grass we've so kindly cultivated for them.

Yes, I know – where I live is hardly typical: kangaroos actually do hop along main roads here. Recently, a friend of mine living further from the bush than me found an echidna in her backyard. It's pretty special; I know I'm privileged. But take heed, humans: we can all have this. We can, we can. And we need it – we can't go it alone.

1 June

It's officially winter now. Three weeks until the shortest day of the year, but not the coldest. Did you know it's often colder after the winter solstice? It takes a while for the earth's deep warmth to dissipate, and even as the days are lengthening there's a similar lag before the earth gathers heat again.

I enjoy this time when the days are closing in and the cold is here to stay. It's as if I've been given permission to look inwards. To step back from things for a while.

Yes, it's true I've been doing that for over a year and a half now, but this feels different. My head is clearing, my body is growing stronger – even if at a snail's pace.

When I was young, I imagined there was a real me who just needed locating. (There she is – isn't she great?) Once found, I'd be this true person who made sense. To be honest, I never really stopped believing that until…you know. Cancer Kate came along.

Is this a blinding revelation? No. But it's kind of entertaining.

Let me start with Tamoxifen. It's over six months since I last swallowed a pill and I can still feel its effects. Mostly in those wobbly moments of gloom before rising. Or when a tidal wave of hopelessness crashes over me, convincing me that I'm useless, washed up and pathetic beyond imagining. Tamoxifen has this way of digging out my deepest darkest fears, my most shameful emotions, and burying me in them.

In the past, I knew these feelings and sometimes felt their hot breath, but rarely got burnt. More and more, that is again who I am.

I'm returning to my own peculiar brand of weirdness. Yay, she's back! But who is she?

Ah, back to my point.

I am a chemical creature – sometimes heartbreakingly so. By now I've made that pretty clear. The food I eat, the chemicals I put in my system or that find their way in, and the chemicals my body manages – hormones, neurotransmitters and more – they all affect me. But I'm more than chemicals: I'm a cloud of energy and atoms influenced by… pretty much everything.

We all know how the weather influences us and, perhaps less so, the earth's energy fields around us. Some places are invigorating, others heavy and lifeless. We don't know why, we just feel it. Then there's people. Whether we notice or not, we're all affected by the energy of others. Think of the people we love to be around, and the ones who make us cringe. Some people bring out the best in us, others the worst.

I feel like one of those Magic 8 balls that you shake and it gives you an answer. Shake me today and receive 'signs point to yes'. Tomorrow, 'reply hazy, try again'. Or my favourite: 'cannot predict now'. Yep, that pretty much sums things up. There's no standard, no yardstick at my centre. Who I am changes, day by day. I'm cool with that. For today at least.

10 June

On the weekend, I cleaned some algae out of the fish tank, looking for Hope. When I found her little body behind a rock, I wanted to cry. She was such a feisty little survivor. Why now?

I buried her in the garden with a generous sprinkle of fish food to keep her going in the afterlife. No more fending off Top Dog Guppy, I told her with a smile. I covered her grave with one of the last camellia flowers, and thanked her for spending her time with us.

Her death feels symbolic, but I'm unsure which way to see it. Is it a bad thing, the death of Hope? But no, death takes us all. She lived longer than most of her kind: surviving the fish plague and a nasty growth, outliving a string of bullies.

When we have hope, we're looking forward. Keeping ourselves open to life's possibilities. That's a marvellous thing.

16 June

A year ago, I went for my thirtieth radiotherapy treatment. As Linac 2 scorched me with its invisible rays one last time I counted down the seconds, preparing for my release. The warning lights clicked off, the room lights came on and a technician bustled in. Done. My active treatment was over – I was through.

Before I could leave, a nurse checked the hot square of skin over my breast and underarm, and exclaimed about how good it was looking. (Some people end up with blisters and burn dressings; lucky me.) She reminded me that I'd probably feel worse for the next couple of weeks, but given how well I was coping she was sure I'd be fine.

Then over to see my radiologist, who also complimented me on my red-but-not-too-red skin. I asked why my muscles felt so terrible and she explained that my damaged skin cells were stimulating the release of cytokines. These chemicals are involved in the healing process and bring on flu-like symptoms (tiredness, achy muscles) which signal the need to rest. She gave me one of her lovely, beaming smiles. 'All normal – now it's time for a well-earned break. And you'll be starting on Tamoxifen soon, won't you? Good, good – but no need to worry about that for a little while, hmm?'

So I left. The automatic doors slid closed behind me and I was outside, blinking in the cold winter light.

*

Back then, I imagined I'd need a month – two, max – to recover from radiotherapy. It could take a bit longer to adjust to Tamoxifen, which I was due to start taking in early July, so I reckoned by September or October I'd be much better.

A year on, post Tamoxifen, here's my tally: I'm low on energy; my muscles are weak and my joints stiff and easily strained; my fingers still go numb after some activities; my moods are erratic; my right arm has lymphoedema and my left has damaged veins; my breast and underarm are still sore…

Who'd have thought?

But here's another tally. Breast cancer? No! Alive and kicking? You bet.

17 June

Here's something to put a cat among the pigeons. In May 2015, an article in *New Scientist* ('Ommm…aargh!') reported that it's not uncommon for people to suffer adverse effects from meditation such as elevated stress levels, panic or depression. The gist of the article is that meditation and similar practices are powerful tools but not always beneficial ones: while some people may feel relaxed and mentally calm, others may end up distressed. Furthermore, it suggests that believing these practices will transform your life is simplistic because in essence they are designed to promote a sense of detachment rather than self-realisation. Food for thought…

What also got my attention in the article is the implication that unearthing negative feelings and thoughts isn't necessarily a good thing. This challenges the thinking that unveiling our inner demons is therapeutic – something I've been mulling over for a while (in case you hadn't noticed). Can you really 'get over' negativity just by exposing it?

Here's what I think. We've developed the ability to store physical and emotional memories for a purpose: they help us stay alive. The more information we gather about our environment, the better. It's particularly important to pay attention to anything that can hurt us – which in our sophisticated human world is not just obvious physical threats like wild animals or poisonous foods, it's also the emotions of others. Emotions are useful tools: we humans use them to protect the social unit. We reward good social behaviour with positive emotions, and we use negative emotions to make individuals toe the line or to punish those who threaten the community's survival.

What I'm getting at is that people's negative emotions can be nearly as damaging as physical threats. If we're ostracised by our community, we can end up alone in a dangerous world. That may be less problematic in our modern world, but in a primitive setting you won't last long if you're booted out from the tribe.

So whether we're aware of it or not, negative emotions tag our memories, lying dormant until they're needed to jump out and warn us. Just like the memory of pain, which engraves itself in our bodies so next time we find ourselves in a similar situation the memory resurfaces. Stop! Be careful! (Like me in the Grampians.)

I guess it's not surprising that when we use techniques to unearth long-buried memories or emotions, the result can be overwhelming.

But is it beneficial to do this? To answer that, we need to solve two problems.

First, is it bad to hang onto intense feelings if they're protecting us from future harm? The trick is to know when the memory of harm is more damaging than the possible harm it may be protecting you from. As an example, let's go back to my memory of being trapped in a sleeping bag by my older brothers (uh oh, getting personal again). I didn't know for sure that it was just a game – all I knew was that I couldn't breathe easily and despite my cries they wouldn't let me out. Maybe I would die! Now of course I know they didn't want to hurt me, they just wanted to scare me. (Ah, the world of children.) But say I'd ended up with severe claustrophobia from such an event, enough to stop me getting in airplanes or lifts or perhaps even cars? Then the emotion attached to the memory is harming me more than it's protecting me.

What about the memory of an intense trauma like a horrific accident? It depends on how protective the memories are – if you live in a war zone and the chances of something terrible happening again are high, then you need that self-protective anti-trauma response. However, if the risk of the event recurring is low and you have detrimental phobias and behaviours because of the trauma, there's definitely an argument for trying to dampen the memories.

This leads on to the second problem. Does the process of reliving memories and feelings actually set them free? In my experience, not really. And why should it? The memories are there for a reason – lessons from our past to guide our futures. But as I've already explained, sometimes these memories are more harmful than helpful. And there are some techniques which do seem to rob memories of their emotional power. For example, you can treat people with serious phobias by gradually helping them face their fears (memories) in a protected way. Mind you, I'm no trauma expert, so remember this is just me mulling over things.

In my long-winded way, I'm getting around to this. While simply exposing negative memories probably doesn't change anything, it is possible to calm them by overlaying them with less stressful ones – a kind of emotional retraining.

Mindfulness does this by observing the memory/emotion and letting it be – which somehow drains the intensity from the feeling, lets it come adrift somewhat. When I try this, I find myself less involved in my emotions, and it opens the possibility of changing them if I want to. It's fascinating actually.

In the same vein, here's another technique I learnt several years ago. Basically you relax by breathing deeply and then take yourself back to a stressful event or feeling and immerse yourself in it. Let the emotions fill you, breathe them in until they peak, then start to surround them. Contain them within a ball which you can now begin to push away. As the ball leaves your body, start to shrink it and squash it until it's just a tiny disc then blow it away. Blow HARD, be gone! Now take yourself back into your stressful place and see how you feel. You'll be amazed.

But clearly these sorts of techniques are much more difficult when remembering traumatic situations where you can be swamped by emotions and unable to contain them. I'd say most of us are a veritable minefield of buried emotions, so it's no wonder even simple meditations can lead to unexpected consequences.

And really, it seems to me that some things are better left alone.

Let's not forget too that negative memories are not always bad for us. Like grief. Why would you want to negate the depth of feeling once felt? If I've experienced grief, won't that make me more likely to step forward when I see someone else at risk? And doesn't the memory of my grief make me less likely to inflict the same on others?

18 June

Some things are better left alone. How true is that?

It reminds me of a movie I saw a few months back called *Wild*. It's a true story based on an emotionally damaged woman who treks across America in a kind of quest – more to escape her past than to find herself. As she traverses hostile desert, snow-capped peaks and finally verdant forests, the audience slowly learns what happened to scar her so.

At the end, there's no Hollywood-style resolution – only this: 'Let it be.' Just that. The woman accepted her demons and left them alone. She moved on. I loved it.

21 June

Today is the winter solstice – an occasion to celebrate, methinks. Not that I'll do anything this time. (But maybe when I'm older I'll drag my witchy drapes out of mothballs and dance around a bonfire each year.) Despite deepening winter cold, the solstice reminds us that the sun is now spending just a little longer each day warming the earth.

I'm always amazed by how quickly some plants respond to the lengthening daylight hours. The bulbs in our back garden emerge ridiculously early, bright green tips of life so foolishly optimistic in the frost. And the wattles out front burst into action while the winds are still blowing off the snowfields – warm golden blooms full of the promise of spring.

1 July

The year is powering along. Already nine days past the solstice and moving towards spring. Well, not quite – last night we had a cracker frost and it can't be more than 5°C outside right now.

Over the last few weeks, I feel like I've been bunkering down. Not in a bad way – more as if I'm coasting, watching the world, resting. Everything feels finely balanced – but also easily damaged. So I've been pulling back, engaging less, being gentle with myself.

Some days, I wonder if I'm in some sort of delayed shock. I started part-time work last September, when I was still recovering from radiotherapy and Tamoxifen was beginning to drag me down. When I stopped Tamoxifen in December, it took months before I felt the fog really lifting. But it was only when my work ran out in early May that I had time to stop and look around.

Which is where I'm at now. In this strange, drifting state. It's not unpleasant; it may even be a good thing.

I know this time can't last. I need to get some work and start making plans for my (better) future. Yes, yes, I will. Soon.

8 July

It's possible I'm boring everyone around me ('Get over it, woman!') but I have to say this. The effects of my treatment just go on, and on, and on...

Over the last few weeks, I've played a few games of squash to test myself out. Surprisingly, I've found myself to be fitter than I thought, fast on my feet, and as competitive as I ever was. Not that I'm a fantastic player, but I'm reasonable.

I monitored myself over the days following each game and assessed myself as stiff and sore – but not much more than is usual (it's a tough game). So, in my excitement, I booked in for a comp starting in August.

Yeah, right. Because now the niggling complaints are starting. My right hand's a bit puffy all the time. My left hip hurts after I've been sitting a while. My right ankle feels a bit dicky.

I went to see my osteopath the other day and she said my hip was sore because my pelvis was slightly out of alignment, making the bone stick out more than it should and irritating the muscle passing over it. Worse than that, she spent ages working on my neck and head, and finally announced that the bony plates on the back of my skull were compressed. What the?

She reminded me that it takes the body's cells a long time to recover from chemotherapy and radiotherapy. So while the most active cells are hit hardest (skin, hair, nails, immune system, digestive system), they also repair quickly. The longer-lived cells, although less damaged by chemo, take longer to heal.

This is sadly what I've been realising. All my little physical glitches add up to one biggie: I am structurally unsound. So I'm going to have to pull out of my squash comp ☹.

And there's more. I hadn't noticed until my osteopath pointed it out: my right upper arm is quite noticeably bigger than the left. Turns out the puffiness in my hand is the proverbial tip of the iceberg. So it's back to a lymphoedema specialist for me.

Clearly I need more healing, more time.

20 August

As I type, the fingers on my right hand struggle to span the keyboard, their movement compressed by tight spandex. My hand, my wrist, my whole arm – wrapped in ugly beige. Now I have to wear a compression glove and sleeve for lymphoedema. Another permanence, another broken part of me.

But with the steady sounds of air conditioning and jet engines filling my ears, there's an upside. I'm off to France to see my daughter. Jammed in economy, eyes bleary after a few broken hours of sleep, but still, here I am.

I have hopes for this trip. I want it to lift me from myself, take me from this moroseness that is so pointless. I am alive. It is that simple, isn't it? That's all we have. I've been squandering my time throughout my many years of wishful thinking, and more recently during the extended months of my cancer fallout.

Last month, I had another check-up. A big date in my diary with nothing outcomes. My surgeon is not a magician: she can't see inside me. She's not going to look at me sitting opposite her and say, 'Oh crap, you have cancer again.' A quick examination, a quick summary chat – nothing more.

There will be more of these visits – if I'm lucky, as non-eventful as that.

Time to start looking forward.

15 September

Back on an airplane, this time heading home. Life happens so quickly. Damn.

I won't talk much about the trip, as this was my forgetting cancer time. And I can tell you I did a good job of it…eventually. I'd like to say I breezed through the four weeks like my travelling self of old – confident and on top of things – but never mind. I got there in the end.

Here's a day which encompasses what I'm talking about. We were staying in the tiny village of Chateauneuf-de-Chabre, near the Gorges de la Méouge in south-eastern France. We'd spent the morning in nearby Sisteron, where the broad river valley narrows abruptly to pass between mountains, and late in the day (after a tea pit stop) we decided to drive from the Gorges de la Méouge up a narrow road to a lookout with views of the gorge and surrounding country.

I was still apprehensive behind the wheel. After thirty-three years of driving on the left side of the road, the switch to the right was completely disorienting. My right hand fumbled with the gearstick, my eyes kept missing the side and rear mirrors, and I couldn't judge the car's position on the road. My daughter was impatient with me – for her, the switch was easy – but I wouldn't let her drive as the insurance costs were too high. So she was stuck with her Nervous Nellie mother.

We took the turn off and drove upwards, enjoying the view of the craggy gorge unwinding below. Then the road narrowed, cutting into the cliffs on our right, while on the left a low rock wall was all that separated us from thin air. Unnerving? Not at first – I was busy convincing myself that this was a one-way road. Then my daughter reminded me that there were no one-way signs. Hmm.

She was right, of course. On this road, even two tiny cars like ours would struggle to pass, but what about a truck and a tiny car? Once the true scariness of the drive was established, my heart began to race and I craned forward in my seat as if those extra few centimetres would save us from a collision. Holy moly.

We rounded bend after bend at a snail's pace, horn blaring, with my daughter alternatingly wincing as I cleared jutting rocks with millimetres to spare, or reminding me I had plenty of clearance so I needed to 'move over!' If I'd been able to turn round and go home, I might well have done so.

At last, the roadsides widened and we drove more gently upwards through thick forest. Much better. A couple more hairy turns, then we cleared the trees and found ourselves on top of the world.

The Table d'Orientation – one of those circular plaques marking points of interest in a 360-degree vista – sat on top of a bare peak with fabulous views all around. To the south east was the town of Sisteron and the citadel that we'd visited that morning, built high on a ridge beside the river pass. This seriously forbidding fort dates back a mere seven centuries or so – not very impressive for an Australian. (Joking! We think a 150-year-old house is ancient.)

A green river valley speckled with farmhouses spanned north from our lookout while all around us high peaks jostled for space. In the foreground, Gorges de la Méouge cut deeply into the limestone, the turbulent river at its centre carting a load of grey sediment southwards to Sisteron and beyond.

It was late in the day and the colours were soft and inviting. The sort of setting where you can't help but lift your arms high and spin in circles. Mountains, forests, valleys, farms, life!

Driving down through the forest, we saw a deer. Or its backside anyway, since it wasted no time bounding off into the trees. And on the downhill run, although I tensed up and craned forward in preparation, somehow the drive was easier. In this direction, I could see that the wall separating us from the abyss had taken more than a few hits from cars, but nonetheless my heart beat slower and my daughter looked slightly less terrified. (And admittedly, no one came in the opposite direction.)

Relaxed and triumphant, I drove us back to our quaint little apartment where leftover curry and a nice red wine awaited us. It was, in the end, a very good day.

21 September

I hoped that going overseas would shake me out of feeling sorry for myself, and remind me that I can be something other than Dreary

Cancer Person. And it worked. With my daughter, I felt fitter and brighter than I had in a very long time.

The timing was perfect, because before leaving I was falling into another depression. Knowing that my lymphatic system was permanently damaged, that my best hope into the future was good management – it was another blow. Just when I was at the point where I could carry off the 'I'm a normal person again' routine, I was given a new badge of dishonour. How many people wander around with their whole arm and most of their hand encased in a beige control garment? Not many.

Anyway, enough of that. I went away and immersed myself in bigger and better things, and now I'm ready to move on.

2 October

Part of moving on involves accepting that more or less is good enough.

Since my return, I've been overdoing things (gardening, mowing, lifting boxes, sweeping up mountains of leaves). My lymphoedema sleeve and gauntlet are intensely irritating because I have to protect them from dirt and damage. If you're someone like me who is clean and tidy, imagine having to don a rubber glove every time you chop onions, stir a spitting pot or wring out a dishcloth.

Because I've been doing too much, my neck problem has flared up – so I'm sleeping badly and my fingertips are doing their numb/tingly thing again. In the mornings, I have to force myself into the shower to wash away the sludginess of my thoughts. But nonetheless, life for me is improving, more or less. And that, my friend, will have to do.

21 October

So, some good news. Yesterday I went for a routine visit to my oncologist. I reminded him of something he'd once said: that the chances of a recurrence are much lower after the two-year mark. 'Two years from when?' I asked him. 'From the end of my treatment?'

'No,' he said, 'from diagnosis.'

Aha! My two years are very nearly up. I'm taking that as a win.

31 October

For Halloween, I bought some lollies: tiny red frogs for any kids who knocked on the door. It was raining and I hadn't put a glowing pumpkin on my doorstep (or whatever you're meant to do), so most of the frogs ended up in my belly.

That's fine. Since my trip away, I've relaxed my standards, just a bit. I drink a little wine now, allow myself a few squares of chocolate – heck, the other day I even bought some Cheezels.

I stuck rigorously to my staying healthy plan (see Appendix) for over six months: it got me over the panic hump when I stopped taking hormonal therapy. And while I'd like to say my diet and lifestyle improvements have made me feel amazing, it seems that, overpoweringly, my damaged body is still in a state of recovery. Slowly, slowly wins the race.

Anyway, my health plan will stand me in good stead into the future. It's a long-term strategy to help me remain cancer-free. And since it's long term, I will add this: over-earnest self-deprivation breeds misery – and a few treats are good for the soul.

4 November

So the Big Day rolls around again. Two years since my diagnosis. Can I start celebrating? Statistically, yes – but emotionally, no. I'll breathe easier after my scans at the end of the month.

Meanwhile, I've come up with some interesting tidbits to tide me along. All my deliberations about why I developed breast cancer keep ending in a fog. My best theory, that an overload of oestrogen was most likely the trigger, still ends with this. What caused the overload?

There's no history of breast cancer in my immediate family. My three older sisters and I grew up in the same environment, ate similar food, did similar activities, but they're all fine. No clues there.

The other day, I was reading about the current shortage of baby formula in Australia, and it got me thinking. I know a lot of mothers have to use formula, but nonetheless isn't it interesting that in our health-conscious society, we're mostly happy to feed babies powdered food? Surely bottle-fed babies miss out on some of the goodness they need?

Then it occurred to me that I was bottle-fed. My mother managed to breastfeed all of her babies until she had twins. Marty and I were too much for her, so we got bottles.

Are bottle-fed babies more prone to breast cancer? A good theory but my rudimentary efforts at research revealed some leads but a shortage of evidence. However, along the way I found in the journal *Breast Cancer Research* (January 2008) a review of breast cancer studies which concluded that twins (particularly non-identical ones like me) may have a higher risk of developing breast cancer. This is because in-utero oestrogen levels are twice as high in mothers pregnant with twins than those with a single baby. Furthermore, being born to an older mother and having a higher birth weight are also factors associated with increased risk.

Where does that leave me? Twin? Tick. Older mother? Tick. Mum was nearly thirty-eight when I was born. Heavy baby? Tick. I was a fatty boomba, hogging the goodies while my skinny brother slunk around on the sidelines. Poor little guy.

Again, this is proof of nothing, but still…

8 November

Remember my story about seeing whales from our apartment balcony at Rainbow Beach last October? A couple of weeks ago down the south coast I saw the most amazing thing. Two humpback whales, maybe three – but definitely at least a female with her baby.

My husband saw them first, one tail and then another rearing up and slamming down like giant hands smacking the ocean. Then came the noise, slightly delayed by distance – the crash of a tail hitting water, echoed quickly by another. Over and over, curving tails to the sky then down. Bang! Bang! Bang! I know I'm overdoing the descriptions but it's not something you see every day. I've never seen such a display.

We wondered if something was wrong, but it seemed not. The

whales kept up their performance with only occasional pauses, slowly moving southwards until they disappeared around the headland.

My two friends (who were staying with us) and I pulled on shoes and hurried along the track towards the point. We could hear the whales on the other side now, still slapping the water. When we reached the top of the south-facing cliffs, there they were again, the water frothing white around them. Bang, bang, bang.

Was this a lesson for the baby whale? A warning system for other whales? Mr Google suggests it may be to remove parasites, or a display of aggression, or in humpbacks a technique for scaring fish into tighter schools prior to feeding.

Or maybe, they were just having fun. Life can't be easy for whales, so why wouldn't they indulge in a bit of entertainment to relieve the burden? Surely this sort of behaviour isn't just a human thing.

The other day I saw *The Martian*, a movie about an astronaut who gets left behind on Mars (presumed dead). I know plenty of people consider space exploration to be a serious matter but during the movie I decided that it's largely a form of escapism. Life on earth can get pretty heavy; why not distract ourselves by trying to solve the great mysteries of our universe? In the movie, NASA and China's CNSA go to great lengths to rescue the astronaut, who has been left trying to grow potatoes inside a flimsy shelter. They get him, of course, after a series of increasingly improbable events. If such a scenario actually occurred, would we spend all that money rescuing one person in space? I think yes.

Stories like that lift us from our humdrum existence. Blasting rockets into space in search of bigger, better worlds? Yeah, baby, let's do it. Creating stories where people pull out all stops to protect a good guy who has been left in an unimaginably terrifying situation? Worth every penny for that warm buzz of achievement, of something better out there than going to the office every day and mowing lawns on weekends.

We need escapism. We need fun. And maybe one day we'll discover a giant water-filled space submarine cruising around Pluto filled with – you guessed it – humpback whales.

26 November

I seem to be coming to the end of this tale. Girl triumphs over breast cancer and lives happily ever after? Yeah! Well, here's hoping.

Time to tie up some loose ends.

My lymphoedema story is improving. The ugly compression garments are doing their job and I'm working towards wearing them less and less. For now, I'm trialling every second day, and hopefully in time I'll only need them occasionally (when doing activities that cause swelling). Unfortunately, those unnoticed months of having a slightly puffy arm have caused some changes: my upper right arm is flabbier than the other, and this is probably permanent. But most likely I'm the only one who'll ever notice.

Despite my continuous ups and downs, overall I'm still improving. I don't feel like my usual self, but when I tell people this they smile and remind me that I'm nearly fifty so I can't expect too much. Damn, I'm already consigned to the old-age scrap heap.

I know I haven't talked about energy fields for a while now, but I feel the need to round off that topic too. I started down that road wondering if my body would reveal a key event that triggered the whole chain of events. 'You got cancer because you're damaged and sad, and it all started with…(insert damaging, saddening event/s).'

Well, no, that theory is just too simplistic. Everything's connected and emotions have their role to play, but I'm not ready to label my emotions as the cause. A contributing factor maybe, but I'm not allocating percentages ☺.

Anyway, that's no excuse for neglecting my emotional energy. So, time to lie down and breathe…

There. Across my shoulders and down both arms – a fat yoke like carthorses wear, heavy and bearing down. This is the legacy of my damaged arms: lymphoedema on the right, scarred veins on the left. As I breathe into the yoke, it slowly lifts and my shoulders and arms relax and let it go. My neck is rigid like a mannequin's, propping up a shiny head with a featureless face. (Baldness, facelessness – becoming a disease more than a person.) My neck's been working hard to help me hold my head high. Breath by breath,

I blow life into the mannequin – and whoosh, my face and hair are back. My neck's a bit softer too – but still tentative, on alert. Fair enough.

Now for my breasts. Oh no, the right one black and blue like it's dead, or nearly. Breathing, breathing…and the darkness drains to grey then finally blushes pink. I focus inwards. What's being held in those breasts? A weight of grief and sadness emerges – but no particular event; it's just life. Breathing it away, softly letting it go, and now my upper body's energy is changing to white, pale yellow and then bright like sunshine. That's more like it.

27 November

One more loose end. To finish off this one, I need to go back to the past again.

Rocks. This time they're granite and weirdly eroded. Remarkable Rocks, a jumble of them perched above the cold Southern Ocean. It's school holidays and midwinter. This place really stands out in my mind because of the bizarre, almost macabre way the rocks have been shaped by ocean winds. In my mind I can see my nephew Simeon there, but whether he actually came I'm not sure. It doesn't matter, because he belongs in this memory.

I remember running around with Marty, Mike and Simeon – hiding behind the giant rocks, jumping out and scaring each other, pointing out ghoulish faces in the granite in a further effort to spook each other. Mum begged us to be careful as we ran close to the ocean side where granite dropped towards smashing waves. And just when I'd given up on the hide-and-seek game and settled into oceanic contemplation, I walked past a tall rock curving over like a beak and…

'ROAR!'

The three boys jumped out from behind the rock, laughing their heads off. Ratbags.

Michael must have been terribly affected by Simeon's death – they were closest in age, and I suppose when Simeon was around Mike was relieved of the burden of being the youngest in a huge family. I don't know if my parents talked to Mike about it – he was only fourteen, after all, and emotionally still very young – but certainly I don't remember talking to him much. We didn't do that in our family. It was easier to pretend we were okay.

So, some rocks stay with us. It can't be helped. And who knows which rocks have most weight, or in fact end up having no weight at all?

Like that Edeowie Gorge trip. The day after Michael dropped his pack, we climbed out of the gorge and up the rocky slopes of Mount Abrupt. The top is narrow, with breathtaking outcrops overlooking the pound to the south and an elegant sweep of mountains continuing northwards. We were almost at the top when the storm we'd been watching advance across the plains hit us. The thunder and lightning were intense and we scuttled for whatever cover we could find beneath overhanging rocks.

Back then, I wasn't very good in storms. When lightning ripped the sky above us, I screamed at the thunder hot on its heels. Mike laughed at me, cheeky bugger. Rain pelted the rock above us and dripped coldly onto our shoulders. With the next bout of thunder, I screamed again and leapt sideways, skinning my knee. More smirks.

The storm blew over eventually and we emerged into pattering rain. Lightning skittered across the horizon and thunder growled, as if to mock me. I fumbled in my pack for toilet paper and wiped the blood off my knee, embarrassed. Then I looked up and gasped.

A gleaming rainbow was emerging in the east, the colours gathering intensity with every breath. Then, like magic, another arc formed above it, drawing life from the storm. A double rainbow.

We climbed onto the peak and sat there, happy. Somebody found chocolate Tim Tams and handed them around. Nobody said anything. No need.

The plains glistened with water and the lowering sun caught the leftover storm clouds and bathed them with colour. The rainbows grew ever brighter.

This was a moment made in heaven. Surely this was heaven.

I like to think Michael remembered that moment more than the falling pack. And the embarrassing sister.

30 November

A while ago, I was having afternoon tea with my elderly neighbour, admiring the blooming roses in her front garden and chatting about something nice, I can't remember what.

I was nibbling on a shortbread as Audrey talked, thinking how fit and healthy she is for her age (she's a year older than my parents) when the conviction hit me. I would live to be old like her. I just knew it.

Afterwards, I dismissed the feeling as fanciful – but it's nice to imagine that it's true.

Today I drove to the hospital, counting good signs along the way. Green lights, no hold-ups, cruising all the way. Then, easy as can be, a parking space waiting for me right beside the clinic instead of the usual frustrating drive around and around.

The mammogram hurt as much as ever. The ultrasound took forever. My brain reminded me of all the ways my life would crash if these scans tripped me up.

But they didn't. They were normal.

Thank you, universe.

*

When I look in the mirror, there's a middle-aged woman with short, greying hair and tired eyes. But behind me is a trail of footsteps winding backwards, reminding me that Cancer Kate is not the sum of me.

Appendix

Plan for staying well

I've taken all the bits of info I've dredged up recently and scrunched them together into my forward plan.

It goes like this:
- avoid processed sugar and alcohol
- eat more whole foods and fibre, less red meat
- eat lots of broccoli (especially broccoli sprouts)
- take Vitamin D supplements in winter if needed
- do more exercise, increase oxygen intake
- relax more
- avoid chemicals, especially xenoestrogens.

Yeah, I know, it's not that radical – but for me it's interesting. I should add that I'm not putting this here to be prescriptive or present myself as some kind of breast cancer guru. When it comes to diet and lifestyle, the literature is awash with information and it's hard to know what to believe.

My primary source of diet information is the website foodforbreastcancer.com, which I believe presents detailed and precise information from a range of well documented sources. But it's a full-time job getting to the heart of every issue, so by necessity I've taken the precautionary approach. As I keep saying, I'm hardly in a position to take risks right now. This is my best guess.

Avoid processed sugar

Cancer cells (like all cells) need sugar for energy, but it's an oversimplification to say that sugar consumption fuels cancer. Nevertheless, the indirect links between excess sugar consumption and cancer are strong. Which means it's time for me to step away from the chocolate bar,

Bleak? Tell me about it. Chocolate kept me going through all those months of waking up way too early feeling like crap. I'd sit in bed while the house slept, streaming bad TV shows on my laptop, drinking tea, tucking into giant Toblerone pieces, Bouchée elephants, Lindt Easter bunnies, whatever was in season. And hey – what's a bit of sugar compared to a truckload of chemo drugs and the like?

But I can't take chances now I'm off all treatments. So for now at least, sugar is on my list of no-nos. By this I mean refined (processed) or simple sugars – anything which breaks down rapidly and causes a spike in blood sugar (glucose) levels.

Why? Although there's nothing wrong with glucose in itself – as I said, our cells need it for energy – a chocolate fudge sundae mega-hit is a different story. Those regular blasts of concentrated sugar are bad news, as they play havoc with blood sugar and eventually with insulin levels. While diabetes and obesity are a couple of obvious outcomes, in breast cancer terms high sugar consumption can raise circulating oestrogen levels and is associated with increased breast density (both, as I've already discussed, known BC risk factors).

The best glucose sources for our bodies are the complex sugars or carbohydrates found in unprocessed foods. These break down slowly, providing a steady blood glucose supply, and come packaged with lots of lovely nutrients and fibre.

The sugar story is much more complicated than the breast cancer angle I'm coming from, but it all boils down to the same mantra. Whole foods are better foods.

Moving on, moving on…

Avoid alcohol

Jeepers creepers, how boring can I get? Like high sugar consumption, alcohol can raise oestrogen levels and is associated with increased breast density. There are many studies linking breast cancer with alcohol consumption, and while there's debate over the level of risk, I'm not in a position to test it out.

Mind you, I continue to doubt that alcohol was a factor in my cancer equation. Remember how I was showing signs of high oestrogen levels in my early twenties? Back then, I only drank occasionally and on those occasions never had more than two or three drinks. (Just putting it out there.)

But one must be sensible and precautionary, eh? And so (sniff) this is another thing it won't hurt me to go without.

Eat more whole foods

Definitely a no-brainer. We have evolved over hundreds of thousands of years to eat the food that nature provides for us. And yet even in my shortish lifetime, processed (altered) foods have been taking up more and more space in wobbly supermarket trolleys the world over. We've gotten greedy – going straight to the good stuff: fat, sugar, protein and salt – while neglecting the whole suite of nutrients more natural foods supply.

Don't get me wrong. Hand me some Cheezels and I'll eat 'em. Mmm. But what exactly are they? Does anyone know? Don't tell me it's cheese and corn, because I won't believe you.

I'm not planning to be a food militant, but it's pretty simple. My body needs all the help it can get, and a bowl of Cheezels just won't cut it. And besides, if you start researching the substances in natural foods with anti-cancer properties, you'll be busy for a very long time.

Eat more fibre

Easy. As long as I eat a variety of whole foods to get plenty of both soluble and insoluble fibre, I'm sorted. But let me explain why fibre is important.

As any breakfast cereal advertisement will tell us, fibre helps start our day. With a healthy, um…elimination. In BC terms, bowel movements remove harmful oestrogen metabolites from our systems, so the more regular they are, the better. Fibre also helps stabilise blood sugar levels and reduce inflammation. (Prolonged inflammation in the body as a result of an overactive immune system is implicated in any number of auto-immune diseases, such as arthritis, asthma, irritable bowel syndrome and Alzheimer's disease. Chronic inflammation is also believed to be a factor in some cancers.)

And as I've already said, foods rich in fibre (whole foods) tend to be rich in a whole suite of cancer-fighting goodies. At which point, I'll add a disclaimer. If you like to start your day with a bowl of nicely packaged processed grains, sugar and salt with some bran and vitamins thrown in, go for it. But call it what it is: junk food with fibre added.

Eat less red meat

This one's contentious, but I'm not waiting for the arguments to die down. A number of naturally occurring substances in red meat – particularly well done or fried meat – are linked with breast cancer, along with the growth hormones sometimes fed to livestock. There are also associations between high animal fat intake and breast cancer. Processed meats like bacon, sausages and smallgoods are definitely worth avoiding because of their preservative and fat content, and because they are often fried, producing mutagenic compounds such as HCA (heterocylic amines) which are known carcinogens.

Interestingly, chicken seems to be okay. In fact, some studies link poultry consumption with a reduced risk of breast cancer. However, avoid chicken that's deep-fried or grilled/barbecued with the skin on, as it can also contain those HCAs I mention above. And it's best to eat free-range organic because chickens fed pellets derived from soy products have raised levels of oestrogen in their flesh and particularly fat.

Eat lots of broccoli

Ah, now we get to the interesting bit.

As I've already explained, an excess of oestrogen is a problem for modern women. Even after menopause, when women stop producing oestrogen in their ovaries, they continue to produce it in their fat. (This is an indirect process: the adrenal glands produce androgens, which are converted to oestrogen by the aromatase enzymes produced in fatty tissue. Aromatase inhibitors – the hormonal therapy drugs I'm supposed to be taking – work by interfering with this process.)

So where do all women have fatty bits? Yes indeed, the breasts. Furthermore, as women age, their breast fat cells tend to produce more oestrogen. This means after menopause women have lower circulating oestrogen levels and higher localised levels in their breasts – right in the danger zone.

Since I'm slim and my boobs are small, you'd think my body wouldn't be awash with oestrogen, but clearly this didn't sway my oncologist when he recommended I go on hormonal therapy. So, now I'm off the drugs, I need a strategy to help manage oestrogen levels in my body.

A chance conversation with the woman who owns my local health food store set me in the right direction. As it turns out, the oestrogen story is much more complicated than I realised.

For starters, there are actually three main forms of oestrogen – oestradiol, oestrone and oestriol. Circulating levels of these vary depending on stage of life. However, the one which dominates throughout women's reproductive years is oestradiol, mostly produced in the ovaries. Oestradiol is the big girl in oestrogen-land, with the strongest oestrogenic activity in the body. At the other end of the scale is oestriol, which has a much weaker oestrogenic activity. (The 'strength' of oestrogenic compounds depends on how well they induce oestrogen-like effects when they latch onto cell oestrogen receptor sites.)

With all forms of oestrogen, the stronger the oestrogenic effects, the higher the risk of developing an oestrogen-related cancer. However, it's not just an overload of oestrogen itself that can be a problem, it's also the metabolites produced when oestrogen is broken down in the liver. It's complicated, but basically oestradiol is converted to oestrone, which breaks down into various metabolites. These include two main forms: 16 alpha-hydroxyestrone (16OH) which is a potent oestrogen and 2-hydroxyestrone (2OH), a weak oestrogen. What's interesting is that the body's use of these 16OH and 2OH metabolic pathways isn't fixed, and can be influenced by lifestyle. Poor diet, being overweight, too much alcohol or exposure to synthetic oestrogens or xenoestrogens (oestrogen-mimicking chemicals) can shift metabolism towards the more harmful 16OH pathway, causing excessive oestrogenic activity.

But here's the good news: you can correct the balance. Apart from avoiding the risk factors above, nature has supplied a neat solution. You know how your Mum always said, 'Eat your broccoli, it's good for you,' and you groaned and said, 'Phooey'? Well, Mum was right. Cruciferous vegetables (broccoli, cabbage, Brussels sprouts, cauliflower, kale, bok choy, mustard and so on) contain key nutrients known to shift oestrogen metabolism towards the more beneficial 2OH metabolic pathway.

Furthermore, these nutrients are found in very high concentrations in broccoli sprouts (three to four-day-old broccoli plants). So all you need is some broccoli seeds, a sprouting container and lots of patience – which clearly I don't have since my efforts were short-lived. Also, despite my love of broccoli, I found the sprouts to be less savoury than expected. So I've another solution…ta da – broccoli sprout powder! The taste is no better but it can be downed in a gulp when mixed with juice. The brand I use is organic and has been carefully processed to preserve the active ingredients. (It is effectively freeze-dried sprouts. Stay away from products containing concentrated extracts from broccoli.)

So far, I haven't found much advice regarding the best amount to take, so I stick to a teaspoon a day – roughly equivalent to a quarter of a punnet of fresh sprouts. (I'm cautious with all supplements, and this seems like a feasible amount.)

Just to be sure, I also eat plenty of those yummy cruciferous vegies listed above (lightly cooked is best). Go, girls. Get crunching.

Manage vitamin D levels

We all know about vitamin D – it's the sunshine vitamin. But what's less known is how important it is. Vitamin D is vital for bone health and strengthening our immunity, among other things, and in cancer terms it's thought that calcitriol (the active form of vitamin D in the body) may kill cancer cells and protect healthy cells from DNA (gene) damage. Even more interesting, there's evidence calcitriol suppresses aromatase activity, and if you remember my earlier ramblings, you'll know that aromatase is needed to convert androgens into oestrogens.

No problem, we get vitamin D from the sun, right? As you sit inside reading this, have a think about how much sun exposure you actually get. Australia is one of the sunniest nations on earth, and surely one of the most well-protected. Kids are swaddled against the sun with rashies and flapcaps and sunscreen from ear to ear. Pale skin is in, sunburn is out. And vitamin D deficiency is on the rise. It's never simple, is it? The trick is to get some sun but not too much.

Science nerd that I am, I've always been suspicious of the chemicals in sunscreens (don't get me started), and also questioned the need to use sunscreen all year round. I didn't make my kids wear hats in winter, or every time they walked out the door in summer. So I've hardly been a role model for the anti-skin cancer lobby. Now it appears my cavalier attitude was partly justified, and since I haven't gotten skin cancer so far, perhaps I'm doing something right.

Nonetheless, my vitamin D levels were on the low end of normal just before my breast cancer diagnosis, although that's not surprising since it was the end of winter. It's hard to get out in the sun when you're working most days and it's dark and bitterly cold by five p.m. Given that I got plenty of sun in the warmer months, I doubt vitamin D had much to do with my breast cancer. However, I can't be complacent.

It's not easy to get enough vitamin D from food sources, so my plan is to rely on sunshine except in the latter months of winter. Why? Because our bodies can stock up on vitamin D by storing it in our fat cells and liver. Aren't we clever little vitamin chipmunks? It's hard to get clear guidelines on how much sunshine is enough (given the ugly bugbear, skin cancer, lurking on the sidelines) but I'm aiming for fifteen minutes of midday sunshine on my arms and face at least every couple of days in winter. If I don't get that, I'll take occasional supplements (and never more than is recommended – vitamin D is fat-soluble and can be toxic in high doses). The rest of the year I reckon I'll be okay because I'm often out in the sun.

And in case you're wondering, in summer I now use invisible zinc sunscreens that don't have nasty chemicals in them. I really don't need to add skin cancer to my repertoire.

Do more exercise, increase oxygen intake

Remember that ABC radio talk by Paul Davies where he hypothesises that cells can turn cancerous in low-oxygen, high-sugar environments? Although I've solved my low iron/oxygen problem, there's no harm in trying to boost my blood oxygen levels. And happily, there's an agreeably natural way of oxygenating the body. It's called exercise – heard of that one? A solution straight from nature. And here's another. Inhale…keep going, keep going…hold it…exhale…empty those lungs…repeat. We all know the routine.

Apart from its oxygen-boosting benefits, regular (moderate) exercise has been shown to increase breast cancer survival. This is thought to be because it reduces inflammation, improves blood sugar and hormone levels, and possibly increases immunity. All good things. On your bike girls. And boys…and me.

Relax more

In my musings thus far I've managed to get confused about the effect of stress on health. My best guess is that while we're adept at handling short term stresses, being consistently stressed over longer periods is deleterious. Is stress a big factor in breast cancer? I don't know. In my case I suspect it helped tip the balance rather than being causative.

Regardless, anything I can do to help me handle life has gotta be good.

Meditation is one approach, but as you'll have gathered I'm not into sitting on a mat in the lotus pose chanting to sitar music as incense smoke fills the room…but whatever floats your boat will do. Me, I prefer mini-meditations: taking time to lie down and breathe, focus my energy inwards and pay attention to what's going on. It's a process of distancing myself a little from the buzzing in my head, and making an effort to calm the tensions in my body.

Avoid chemicals, especially xenoestrogens

This is a huge topic but I'll try keep it simple. In fact, that's the answer: as much as you can, keep it simple. I try not to put synthetic chemicals on my skin, on my clothes and in my mouth. I minimise them in my home and my car.

As I've already discussed, our modern world is overflowing with xenoestrogens – chemicals which mimic the action of oestrogen in our bodies.

Here are some I watch out for:

Phthalates. These are found in cosmetics and toiletries (they help the fragrance to 'stick'), in food containers and wraps (PVC plastics, clingwrap, and so on – where they leach into foods, especially fatty products), and in many other soft plastic products.

BPA and PCBs. Bisphenol A (BPA) is used in some plastics and epoxy resins. It's commonly found in plastic drink bottles and as a lining for cans to prevent the contents contacting the metal. Many polycarbonate (PCB) plastics contain BPA – these are clear, hard plastics with many uses including for water and baby bottles.

Parabens. These are used as preservatives in cosmetics and toiletries, and are readily absorbed through the skin. They're also found in pharmaceuticals and some foods.

There are plenty of other xenoestrogen sources to be wary of – they're found in cleaning products, paints, flame retardants (furniture, clothes, car upholstery, and so on), pesticides, herbicides – you could go crazy thinking about it. I avoid the ones I can, and try not to think about those I can't.

The synthetic oestrogens found in the pill or hormone replacement therapy also fit into the xenoestrogen category, but I don't have to worry about them now (apart from the ones women pee out into the environment – true, I'm afraid). And I'm not going to start telling women whether to take them or not, just to be aware of the risks.

*

A note on phytoestrogens

These are naturally occurring xenoestrogens found in some plants. Sources include beans, lentils and other legumes, whole grains and some seeds (for example, linseed, sesame seeds). Phytoestrogens are weakly oestrogenic and are often thought to be beneficial for pre-menopausal women because they occupy cell oestrogen receptors, thereby reducing the effect of the stronger oestrogens in circulation. But high consumption of soybean proteins can mess with women's menstrual cycles, and in my case I've been advised to avoid soy products (because I need to avoid all oestrogen sources…neutering for me, eh?).

Furthermore, I've also read that unfermented soybeans and other legumes contain a range of substances, such as trypsin inhibitors and phytates, which can interfere with protein digestion and the absorption of important minerals like calcium, magnesium, iodine, iron and zinc. Hmm…confusing.

What I think it boils down to is this. Our bodies have evolved to deal with the chemicals in many foods, and heck, if you start reading about the natural toxins found in fruit and vegetables, you'll be busy for a long time. We can cope with these substances in natural form, it's when we start processing and/or concentrating foods that things go awry. My solution is to go back to the basics: a varied diet made up mostly of unprocessed, simple foods is best. If I enjoy a variety of legumes, whole grains and seeds along with many other foods, what's the problem? Legumes are high in fibre and have many health benefits. But a diet tipped heavily in favour of processed soy is another matter.

So it's probably wise to go easy on products like soybean oil, soy protein isolate, tofu and soy milk (icky stuff anyway ☺). And if the Asians have been fermenting soybeans for centuries then, hey, they must know something we don't. Give miso, tempeh and fermented soy sauce a go.

Afterword

This is for my daughters, who I worry have found my story hardest of all. As a mother, I want to present myself as strong, as reliable. Or at least I did – 'cos I've blown it now. It was hard for me to put my frailness and fear on paper for them to read. Here's hoping the biggest messages they take away are to be kind to themselves, to focus on what's right in themselves and the world around them, and remember the lightness and clarity that comes with spending time in nature.

My oldest daughter asked why I wrote so much about a past so far away. University bushwalks, climbing trips in my twenties. She wondered if that meant these were the best days of my life, and that everything had been downhill since. I laughed, trying to frame my answer. It was because back then I had so many ideals. So many expectations of myself and my life. The difference between that girl and old me? Huge. The intervening years were full of life too – not least of which was having babies and helping two miraculous daughters through to adulthood. But the mood of those years was less intensely focused on me. My orbit widened radically – I had less time for inward thinking.

Having cancer gave me time, once again, for myself. Still not sure that was good, but hey, I'll run with it.

This is also for Chico, who died in March 2018 aged fourteen and a half. It was unbelievably sad, not least because of how much he helped me when I was unwell. Early on during my chemo treatment, he started coming into my room every evening and lying on the carpet for a few hours – keeping me company. Eventually the lure of a soft mattress would win out and I'd hear his toenails clicking back down the hallway to his bed. I felt he was looking out for me during bad times.

My chemo started in summer so I assumed that as it grew colder his visits would peter out (given his love of his warm bed). But he kept coming and I grew to depend on him, waiting for the telltale clicking on timber flooring as he approached, enjoying the way he'd come to me for a pat then head for his corner, turn a few circles and flop down with a contented sigh.

He continued with this habit right through until he was too unwell to want to lie on carpet, so instead I started bringing his bed into my room for him. On his last night in this world, I carried him and his bed together, settled him down with a blankie over him even though it wasn't cold, and spent the night listening to his uneven breathing.

I can't tell you how awful his dying was, my friend to the end – I miss you, boy.

www.ingramcontent.com/pod-product-compliance
Lightning Source LLC
Chambersburg PA
CBHW030909080526
44589CB00010B/212